Ulrich Spandau · Zoran Tomic

Small-Gauge Vitrectomy for Diabetic Retinopathy

Second Edition

Springer

Ulrich Spandau
Department of Ophthalmology
St. Eriks University Hospital
Stockholm, Sweden

Zoran Tomic
Milos Klinika
Belgrade, Serbia

https://doi.org/10.1007/978-3-031-26204-3

This Springer imprint is published by the registered company Springer Nature Switzerland AG
The registered company address is: Gewerbestrasse 11, 6330 Cham, Switzerland
(www.springernature.com/mycopy)

Small-Gauge Vitrectomy for Diabetic Retinopathy

Preface

Diabetic retinopathy is the biggest challenge for the VR surgeon. The challenge is twofold; on the one hand, the sheer volume of patients and on the other hand a difficult surgery with a big peroperative and postoperative complication spectrum.

Lack of medical care and the immense volume of patients lead to very advanced cases of a tractional retinal detachment, which untreated often ends in blindness. The vitrectomy of a tractional retinal detachment is the most difficult and challenging ocular surgery. It divides VR surgeons in mediocre and experienced surgeons. Diabetic retinopathy is surgically very demanding because you operate an inflamed and vascular active tissue. The essentials for success are

1. Sequential phaco/vitrectomy
2. Preoperative anti-VEGF
3. Bimanual vitrectomy

We will demonstrate small gauge vitrectomies. We describe the surgery step-by-step. Just like a recipe in a cookbook. First, the ingredients and then step-by-step the preparation. If you follow the recipes you will master this pathology. All steps are visualized with photographs and short videos.

Our endeavour is to teach more people how to master the surgical management of the diabetic eye. We wish every reader, may he or she be a beginner or an advanced surgeon, to enjoy reading this book and watching the surgical videos. All videos of this book are found on the YouTube channel from Ulrich Spandau and playing list "Proliferative diabetic retinopathy" (link: https://youtube.com/playlist?list=PL0dKYclPD7yM9qRjBoF1HMwtxFfbf2T6A).

Stockholm, Sweden
October 2022

Ulrich Spandau
Zoran Tomic

Acknowledgements I am grateful to Dr. Saumya Sanyal for reviewing the manuscript.

Contents

Abbreviations

BIOM	Binocular Indirect Ophthalmo Microscope
C_2F_6	Perfluoroethane, gas for retinal tamponade
CF	Counting fingers
cSt	Kinematic viscosity of a fluid (unit = centiStoke)
HM	Hand movement
IOP	Intraocular pressure
LE	Left eye
LIO	Laser indirect ophthalmoscope
OD	Oculus dexter, right eye
OS	Oculus sinister left eye
OU	Oculus uterque, both eyes
PDVR	Proliferative diabetic vitreoretinopathy
PDR	Proliferative diabetic retinopathy
PFCL	Perfluorocarbon liquid
PPV	Pars plana vitrectomy
PRP	Pan-Retinal photocoagulation
PVD	Posterior vitreous detachment
RE	Right eye
SF_6	Sulphahexafluoride, gas for retinal tamponade
TRD	Tractional retinal detachment

Part I

Essentials for Surgery of the Diabetic Eye

All videos of this book are found on the Youtube channel from Ulrich Spandau and playing list "Proliferative diabetic retinopathy" (link: https://youtube.com/playlist?list=PL0dKYclPD7yM9qRjBoF1HMwtxFfbf2T6A).

Chapter 3.4: Two extreme cases of diabetic retinopathy.

Introduction

1

1.1 Worldwide Facts About Diabetes

(1) The number of people with diabetes increased from 153 million in 2000 to 537 million in 2021. This number is estimated to grow to 783 million in 2045 (International Diabetes Federation 2021, Lancet 2011, WHO 2011)

There is an emerging global epidemic of diabetes that is caused by rapid increases in overweight, obesity and physical inactivity.

(2) The number of people with type 2 diabetes is increasing in every country

Type 2 accounts for around 90% of all diabetes worldwide. Reports of type 2 diabetes in children—previously rare—have increased worldwide. In some countries, it accounts for almost half of the newly diagnosed cases in children and adolescents.

(3) 80% of people with diabetes live in low- and middle-income countries

One hundred seventy-five million people with diabetes are undiagnosed. This is especially the case in the developing countries. The prevalence of diabetes has increased by 150% in developing countries with China and India in the first two positions.

(4) The greatest number of people with diabetes are between 40 and 59 years of age

Diabetes caused 5.1 million deaths in 2013; every 6 s a person dies from diabetes.

(5) Diabetes is a leading cause of blindness

It is estimated that in 2002 diabetic retinopathy accounted for about 5% of world blindness, representing almost 5 million blinds. From being the 20th common

U. Spandau and Z. Tomic, *Small-Gauge Vitrectomy for Diabetic Retinopathy*,
https://doi.org/10.1007/978-3-031-26204-3_1

cause of blindness in 1984 it has become the 6th most common cause of blindness today.

(6) Diabetes is a leading cause of death

Diabetes caused 5.1 million deaths in 2013; every 6 s a person died from diabetes. However, in 2021, it is responsible for 6.7 million deaths, which is 1 death every 5 seconds.

1.2 Regional Facts About Diabetes

Europe: Total population is 740 million and 1 in 11 adults are living with diabetes. The top country for adults with diabetes is Russia with 11 million (absolute number). The top country for prevalence is Turkey with 15% (relative number compared to the total population). Europe has also the highest prevalence of type 1 diabetes in children (Fig. 1.1) (International Diabetes Federation 2021, Lancet 2011, WHO 2011).

Middle East and North Africa: Total population is 370 million and 1 in 6 adults are living with diabetes. The top country for adults with diabetes is Egypt with 7.5 million. The top country for prevalence is Saudi Arabia with 24% (Fig. 1.2).

Africa: Total population is 1100 million and 1 in 22 adults are living with diabetes. The top country for adults with diabetes is Nigeria with 3.9 million. The top country for prevalence is Gabon with 11% (Fig. 1.3).

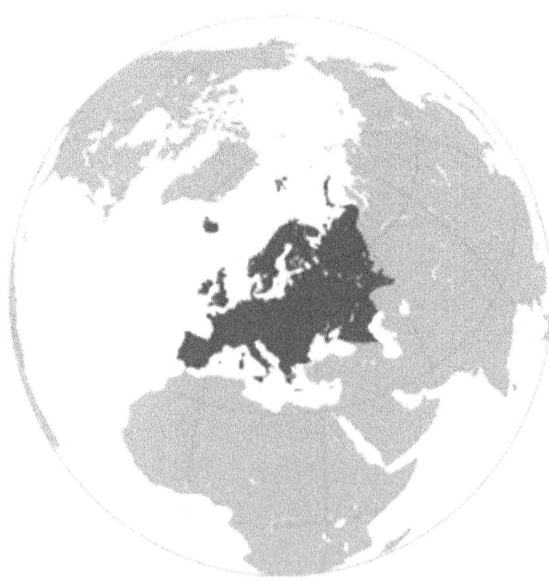

Fig. 1.1 Europe has also the highest prevalence of type 1 diabetes in children. In Europe, Turkey has the highest prevalence with 15%

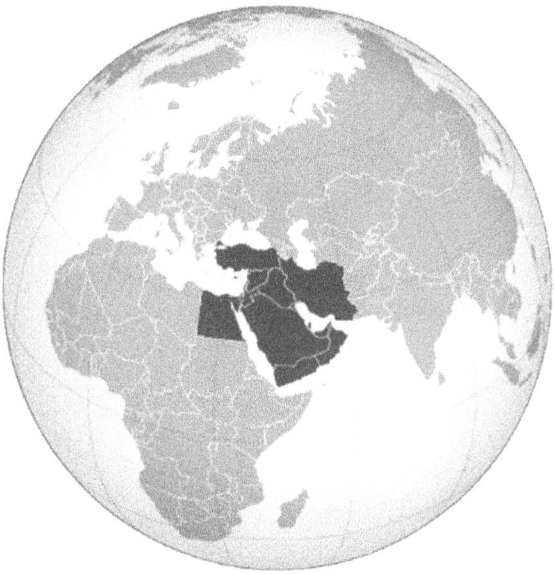

Fig. 1.2 Saudi Arabia has the highest prevalence of diabetes in the Middle East with 24%

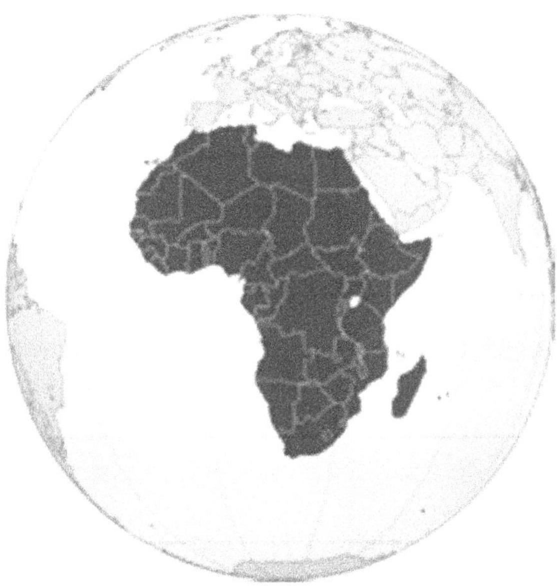

Fig. 1.3 Africa has a fast-growing diabetes population in the cities. Gabon has the highest prevalence with 11%

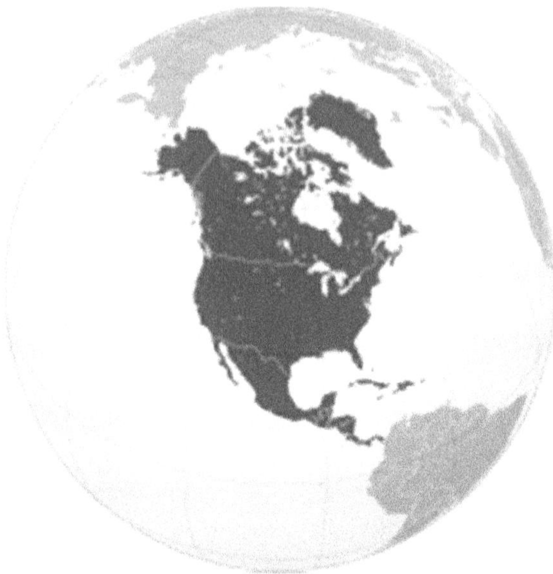

Fig. 1.4 In the US live 24 million diabetic patients. In North America, Belize has the highest prevalence with 16%

North America and Caribbean: Total population is 460 million and 1 in 7 adults are living with diabetes. The top country for adults with diabetes is the USA with 24 million. The top country for prevalence is Belize with 16% (Fig. 1.4).

South and Central America: Total population is 450 million and 1 in 11 adults are living with diabetes. The top country for adults with diabetes is Brazil with 11 million. The top country for prevalence is Nicaragua with 12% (Fig. 1.5). The number of people with diabetes on this continent is growing fast and will increase by 60% until 2035.

Asia: Total population is 4.100 million and 1 in 11 adults are living with diabetes. The top countries for adults with diabetes are China with 98 million and India with 65 million. The top country for prevalence is Malaysia with 11% (Fig. 1.6). However, almost half of the people with diabetes in India and South-East Asia are undiagnosed.

1.3 The History of Diabetic Vitrectomy

The first vitrectomy was performed on an eye with diabetic vitreous hemorrhage. Robert Machemer (1933–2009), the "Father of Vitrectomy", performed his first surgical experiments in 1969 with eggs at the Bascom Palmer Hospital in Miami

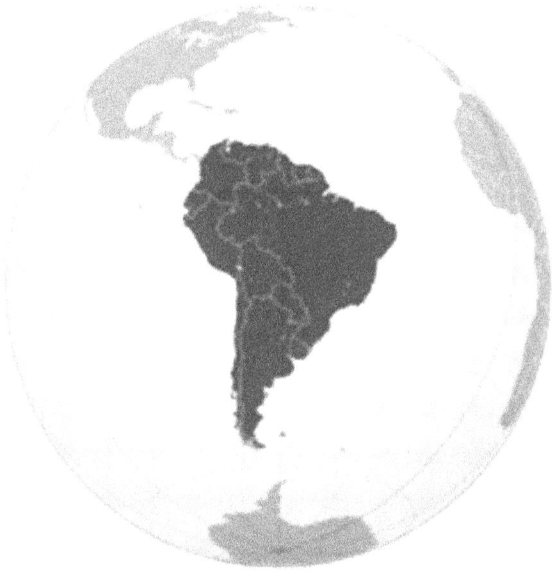

Fig. 1.5 The number of people with diabetes in South America is growing fast and will increase by 60% by 2035

Fig. 1.6 The prevalence of diabetes has increased by 150% in developing countries with China and India in the first two positions

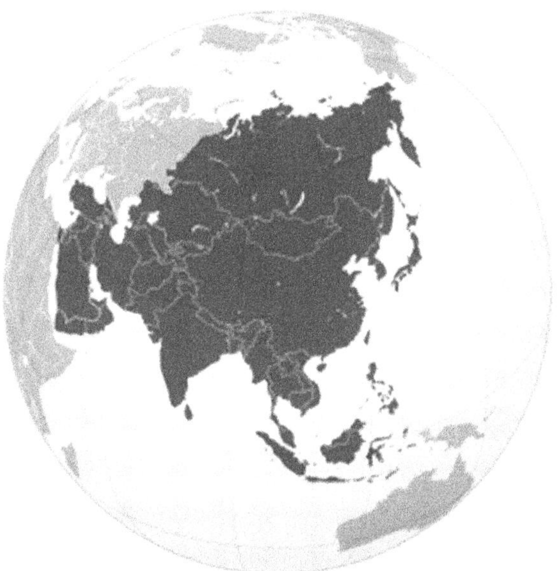

and the first vitrectomies in 1972 (Fig. 1.7). The first vitreous cutter was a 16-gauge (1.3 mm) instrument (Fig. 1.8). The cutting rate was very slow with 1 cut per second.

The most recent development is a 27-gauge vitrectomy (Fig. 1.9). The instruments have a diameter of only 0.4 mm. The small instruments and especially the vitreous cutters which can cut tractional membranes are a "game changer" for surgery of diabetic retinopathy. The cutting rate is 16.000 cuts per second or even higher.

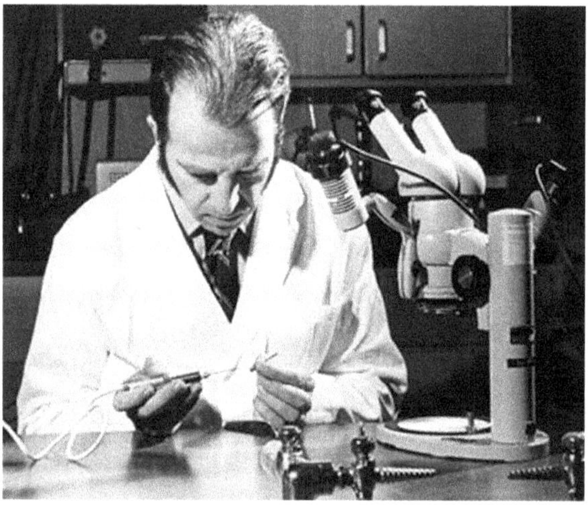

Fig. 1.7 The German-born Robert Machemer is the father of vitrectomy. The first vitrectomy was performed on an eye with diabetic vitreous hemorrhage

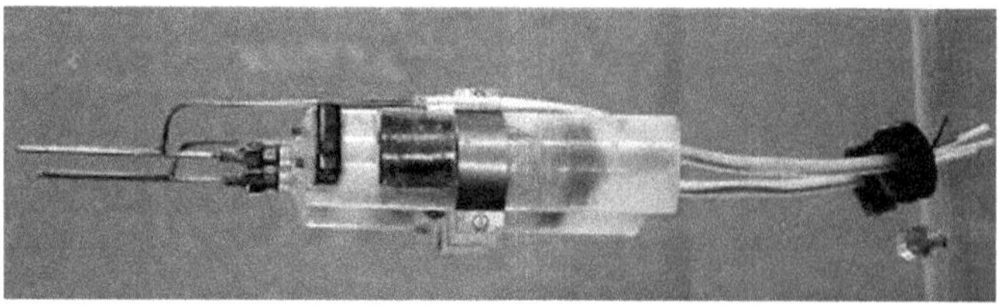

Fig. 1.8 The first 16G (1.3 mm) vitreous cutter

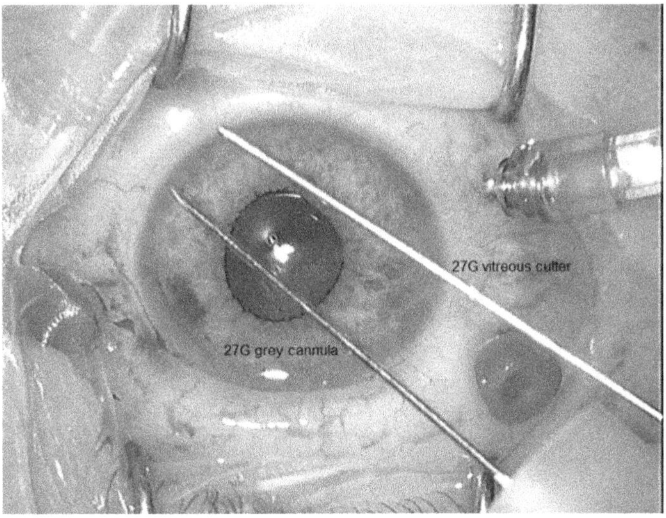

Fig. 1.9 The most recent development is 27G vitrectomy. The size of the 27G vitreous cutter diameter is equal to the 27G cannula

References

International Diabetes Federation. IDF Diabetes Atlas, 10th edn. Brussels, Belgium: International Diabetes Federation; 2021.
Lancet. 2011; 378(9785):31–40.
WHO report; 2011.

Anatomical Pathology of Diabetic Retinopathy

2

2.1 Ischemic Retinopathy

Ischemic retinopathy is an entity of retinal pathologies with the common characteristics of retinal ischemia and **neovascular** proliferations. Untreated, the disease results in a neovascular glaucoma and **tractional** retinal detachment. The most common ischemic retinopathies are diabetic retinopathy, branch retinal vein occlusion (BRVO), central retinal vein occlusion (CRVO) and retinopathy of prematurity (ROP). Diabetic retinopathy and ROP are bilateral diseases whereas BRVO and CRVO occur unilaterally. Less common ischemic retinopathies are familial exudative vitreoretinopathy (FEVR), Coats, Incontinentia pigmenti and many more. Ischemic retinopathy can also be categorized into peripheral and central. Diabetic retinopathy is mostly a central ischemic retinopathy while FEVR and Eales disease (tubercular vasculitis) is mostly peripheral.

The pathophysiology of diabetes is complicated. In short, hyperglycemia triggers endothelial cell dysfunction leading to breakdown of the blood retinal barrier and increased permeability of retinal vessels. The initial pathology is loss of pericytes in the retinal capillaries. The loss of pericytes leads to a defect in the inner blood retinal barrier and a loss of intercellular contact of the endothelial cells leading to the proliferation of the endothelial cells and out pouchings of the capillary wall giving rise to microaneurysms. The glycation of capillary basement membrane molecules (collagen type IV, laminin, entactin, etc.) leads to its thickening. Increased levels of inflammatory cytokines lead to increased leucocyte adhesion to capillary walls by upregulation of adhesion molecules, which further leads to capillary stasis, occlusion and ultimately hypoxia. This hypoxia leads to tissue ischemia which leads to uncontrolled neovascularization in an attempt to compensate for the lack of blood flow. Angiogenesis consists of a series of highly complex biochemical and cellular activity requiring sequential receptor activation by several growth factors such as fibroblast growth factor (FGF), transforming growth factor (TGF), tumour necrosis factor α (TNFα), angiopoietins 1 and 2, erythropoietin (EPO) and

U. Spandau and Z. Tomic, *Small-Gauge Vitrectomy for Diabetic Retinopathy*,
https://doi.org/10.1007/978-3-031-26204-3_2

vaso endothelial growth factor (VEGF). The most important factor among all of them is VEGF. In the retina, VEGF is expressed by RPE cells, neurons, glial cells, ganglion cells, Muller cells, endothelial cells and smooth muscle cells, in response to tissue hypoxia via the hypoxia inducible factor 1α (HIF1α). VEGF induces endothelial cell mitogenesis, induces fenestrations across cell bodies and dissolves tight junction between endothelial cells thereby contributing to leakage and angiogenesis. The eye is the only organ in the human body that forms pathological blood vessels in response to a tissue ischemia. The extent of the retinal ischemia can be best visualized with a fluorescein angiography.

Wide-angle photography and fluorescein angiography are the two essential examinations for diabetic retinopathy for VR surgeons because they reveal the true extent of the retinal ischemia and allow targeted photocoagulation. It is ideal to perform a wide-angle photography (Fig. 2.1) together with angiography (Fig. 2.2) to note the amount of ischaemia and to detect peripheral neovascularization.

Based on the angiography a laser photocoagulation can be planned. A scatter laser has two important effects for a scheduled vitrectomy. Firstly, it reduces the

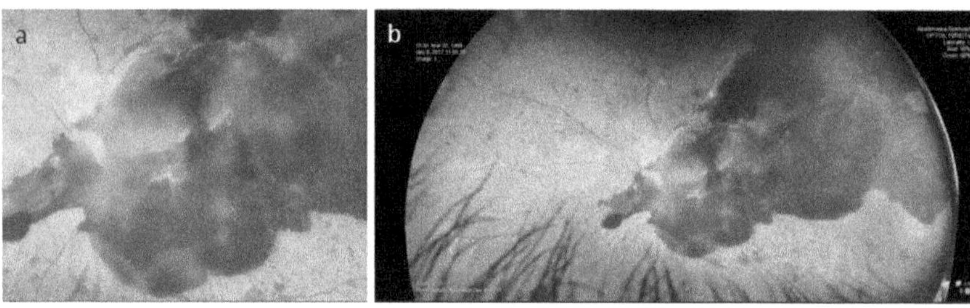

Fig. 2.1 Central pole (**a**) and 270° widefield (**b**) photograph of a large preretinal hemorrhage. The whole extent of the disease is only visible in the widefield photograph

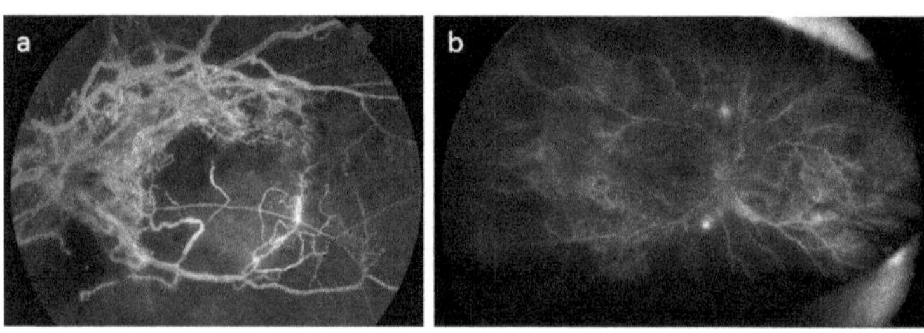

Fig. 2.2 Fluorescein angiography of two different patients. **a** Central field fluorescein angiography showing extensive capillary non-perfusion, leakage from pathological neovascularization and staining of venous walls, all these being consistent with severe retinal ischemia. **b** Optos fluorescein angiography, showing extensive ischemia in the periphery including the retina within the nasal arcade. The temporal arcade is less affected, VA = 0.6

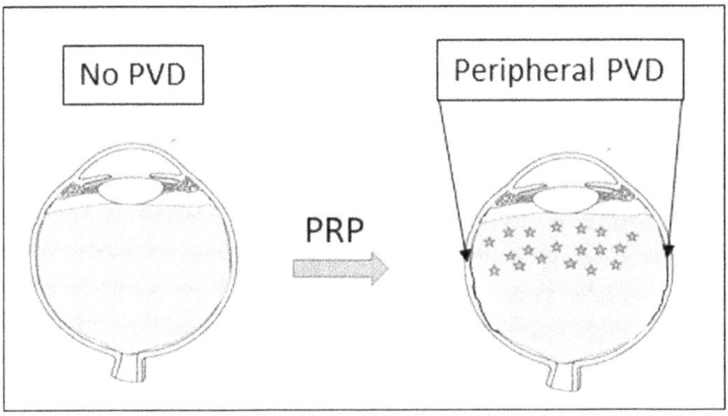

Fig. 2.3 A scatter laser photocoagulation (PRP) induces a PVD. A preoperative PRP facilitates a vitrectomy

grade of diabetic retinopathy and secondly, it induces a peripheral PVD (Fig. 2.3). Please see the double vitrectomy in Chap. 11 "Unusual and difficult cases".

2.2 Anatomical Pathology of a Proliferative Diabetic Retinopathy (PDR)

The three important surgical features of PDR are vitreous hemorrhage, status of posterior hyaloid and fibrovascular membranes.

2.2.1 Formation of Fibrovascular Membranes

Four fundamental pathophysiological processes take place in proliferative diabetic retinopathy [1] 1981:

(1) Proliferation and subsequent regression of new vessels.
(2) Proliferation of fibrous tissue accompanying new vessels. This fibrous tissue is adhesive to the underlying retina. Figures 2.4 and 2.5 show this pathophysiological process.
(3) Formation of adhesions between fibrovascular proliferations and the posterior hyaloid. Figure 2.6 illustrates this process.
(4) Partial contraction of the posterior vitreous with focal detachment. Figure 2.7 shows a drawing of a tractional retinal detachment.

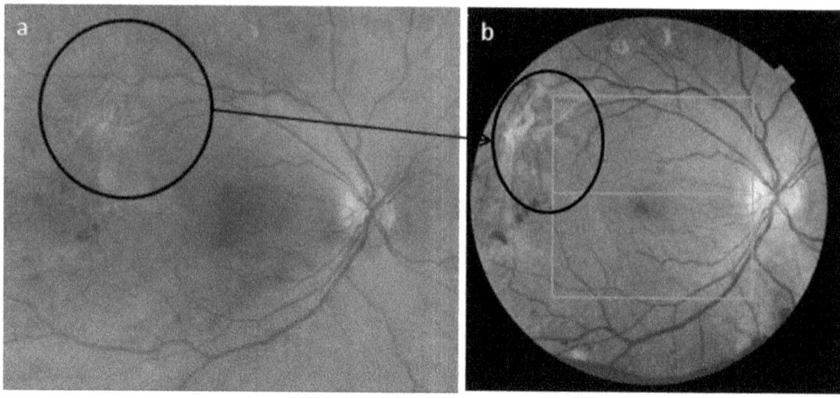

Fig. 2.4 **a** A type 1 diabetic with retinal proliferations at the superior arcade. **b** The same patient one year later. The proliferations have regressed and fibrous tissue has formed

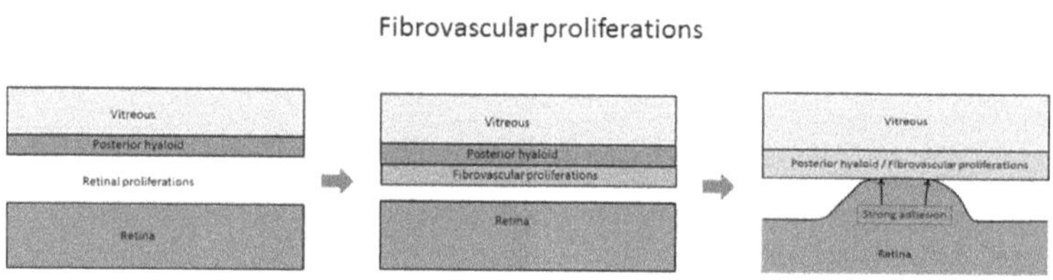

Fig. 2.5 First retinal neovascular proliferations develop which are flat on the retina. Along with it fibrous tissue starts appearing (fibrovascular proliferations) which grows along the posterior hyaloid scaffold. The fibrous component of these proliferations contracts and starts lifting the retina (dynamic traction). Then the retinal proliferations regress and transforms to purely fibrotic tissue (fibrous proliferation). This results in a static traction

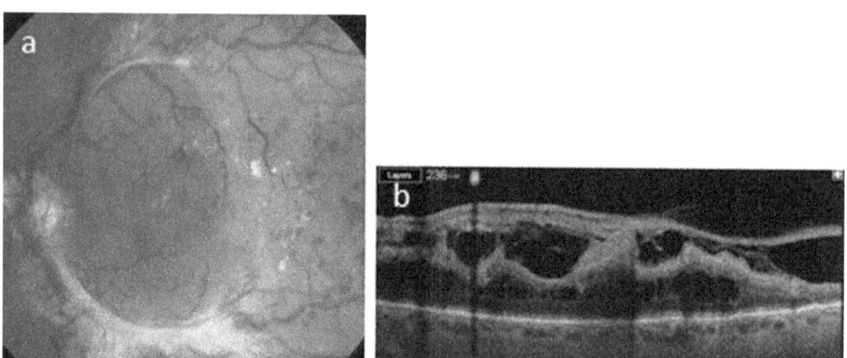

Fig. 2.6 **a** Colour photograph of a severe PDR with fibrovascular membranes. **b** OCT with attached posterior hyaloid and several adhesions between posterior hyaloid and retina

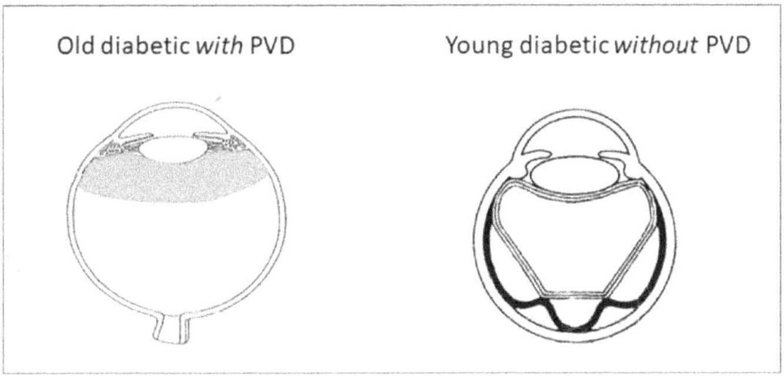

Fig. 2.7 A drawing of the posterior hyaloid anatomy. In an old diabetic a PVD is present, whereas in a young diabetic the posterior hyaloid is attached at the posterior pole

2.2.2 Status of the Posterior Hyaloid

The anatomy of the posterior hyaloid is essential for diabetic vitrectomy (Fig. 2.7). In young diabetic patients, the posterior hyaloid is firmly attached in the centre and periphery. In addition, fibrovascular membranes are attached to the posterior hyaloid. During vitrectomy a complete PVD has to be performed which is challenging because the posterior hyaloid is firmly attached (posterior hyaloid separation), resulting in a difficult vitrectomy. In old diabetics, however, the posterior hyaloid is detached (PVD) resulting in an easy vitrectomy.

2.2.3 Vitreous Hemorrhage

A vitreous hemorrhage is a common phenomenon in diabetic retinopathy. 50% of all vitreous hemorrhages are of diabetic origin. Proliferative retinal vessels are prone to bleeding. The hemorrhage forms first in the subhyaloidal space (Fig. 2.8). The blood cells attach to the posterior hyaloid and stain it. If the posterior vitreous is detached at the posterior pole then the blood can enter the vitreous gel.

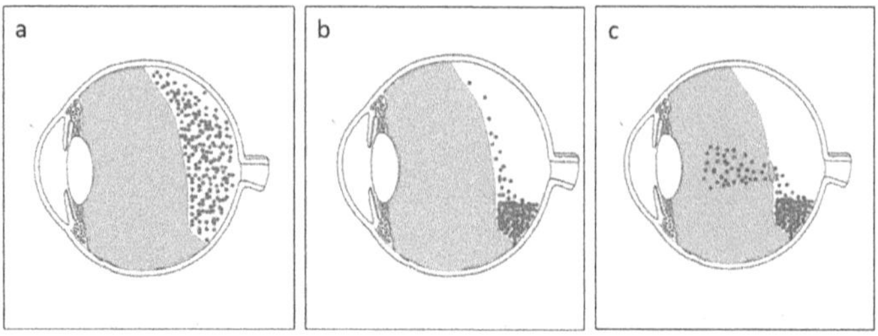

Fig. 2.8 **a** A drawing of a subhyaloidal hemorrhage with impaired visual acuity in a type 2 diabetic. **b** After sleeping with head up the subhyaloidal hemorrhage accumulates at the inferior pole freeing the macula resulting in improved vision. **c** The blood can enter the vitreous gel through the Weiss ring

Reference

Diabetic Retinopathy Research Group. Invest Ophthalmol Vis Sci. 1981; 21:210.

Hot Topics Regarding Vitrectomy for PDR

3

The fear of a negative effect of Avastin is bigger than the fear for a difficult vitrectomy.

3.1 Pretreatment or Not—That is the Question

What are the advantages of a preoperative intravitreal bevacizumab injection?

There is a general consensus to pretreat a diabetic eye with an anti-VEGF injection. What are the advantages of a pretreatment and is it really necessary? A preoperative intravitreal bevacizumab injection results in a significant reduction of vitrectomy times, fewer retinal breaks, less intraoperative bleeding, fewer endodiathermy applications, lowers the incidence of postoperative hemorrhage and last but not least speeds up visual recovery (Arevalo et al. 2019; Smith and Steel 2015).

Duration of surgery. A significant reduction of duration of vitrectomy is associated with preoperative intravitreal bevacizumab (IVB). The reduction in the duration of surgery was between −33 and −18 minutes (Arevalo et al. 2019; Smith and Steel 2015).

Number of intraoperative breaks. The number of intraoperative breaks created during vitrectomy was significantly less in patients undergoing preoperative IVB (Arevalo et al. 2019; Smith and Steel 2015).

Intraoperative bleeding. A significant reduction of intraoperative bleeding is associated with preoperative IVB (Arevalo et al. 2019).

Endodiathermy applications. The average number of endodiathermy applications to control intraoperative bleeding that patients undergoing combined IVB/PPV required fewer endodiathermy applications (Arevalo et al. 2019).

U. Spandau and Z. Tomic, *Small-Gauge Vitrectomy for Diabetic Retinopathy*,
https://doi.org/10.1007/978-3-031-26204-3_3

Postoperative haemorrhage. Patients receiving intravitreal bevacizumab in addition to pars plana vitrectomy had less likely a postoperative hemorrhage compared to patients with vitrectomy alone (Arevalo et al. 2019; Smith and Steel 2015).

Fast visual recovery. Less postoperative inflammation associated with small gauge vitrectomy facilitates early visual recovery in PDR (Arevalo et al. 2019; Smith and Steel 2015).

How long anti-VEGF pretreatment before vitrectomy?

The aim of a diabetic vitrectomy is the removal of the posterior vitreous. Remark: Removal of posterior vitreous implies the removal of fibrovascular membranes along with it. In difficult cases the PVD cannot be induced with the vitreous cutter because the posterior hyaloid is firmly attached to the retina. A forced induction of PVD would result in retinal tears. Therefore, a careful delamination with scissors and forceps is required. Now comes the second problem. If you try to remove the fibrovascular membranes in a not-pretreated eye, then you will experience severe bleedings which are difficult and sometimes impossible to control. Therefore, the retinal bleedings must be suppressed before you perform a diabetic vitrectomy. This can be done with laser and anti-VEGF, ideally with the combination of both. What is the optimal time point of a vitrectomy for a TRD? The answer is when the retinal proliferations are absent. There is a general consensus that a pretreatment with anti-VEGF (and laser) is necessary before scheduling a vitrectomy (Arevalo et al. 2019; Smith and Steel 2015). There is, however, no consensus about the timing. Most surgeons wait 3–5 days (Arevalo et al. 2019; Smith and Steel 2015). A minority waits 2 weeks. We wait 4 weeks (Fig. 3.1). During 18 years of our surgical practice, we experienced only two cases with aggravation of TRD. In one case the macula was not involved so we did not change the planning. In the other case the macula was involved, and we operated immediately. Important: The longer you wait after anti-VEGF injection (maximal 6 weeks) the easier and shorter the vitrectomy becomes because you experience less intraoperative bleeding. The outcome is also better because you experience less postoperative complications such as vitreous hemorrhage and macular edema.

Does anti-VEGF treatment increase tractions in tractive PDR?

An anti-VEGF pretreatment of a diabetic eye with TRD is highly debated within the vitreoretinal society. Anti-VEGF may cause an aggravation of tractions (crunch effect). The anxiety about a crunch effect after anti-VEGF is higher than about a difficult vitrectomy and surgical failure. In our experience, surgical failure is increased if you do not pretreat the eyes. But what does the literature report?

A study by Arevalo et al. first raised potential safety concerns with regard to TRD when intravitreous anti-VEGF agents were used in eyes with PDR (Arevalo et al. 2008). Among 211 eyes with PDR that underwent vitrectomy and received 1.25-mg bevacizumab as a preoperative adjuvant therapy, 11 eyes showed later development or progression of TRD. This is an incidence of 3.5%. But without a

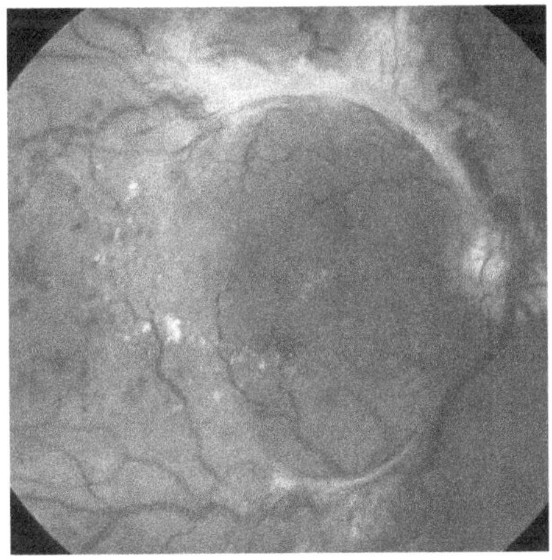

Fig. 3.1 A severe proliferative diabetic retinopathy with fibrovascular membranes on the temporal arcades. This eye we would definitely pretreat with anti-VEGF and wait 4 weeks before surgery. Untreated you will experience severe bleeding during and after surgery

control group, the study design could not rule out the possibility that the TRDs were a result of the natural history of the disease.

Bressler et al. conducted a large prospective study with a control group (Bressler et al. 2020). Patients with PDR and DME were treated with anti-VEGF. The control group received no treatment. All eyes were followed up for 1 year. The results showed that anti-VEGF does not increase the risk for TRD. The risk for TRD is the same in the treatment and the control group. This means that the natural course of the disease and not anti-VEGF is responsible for an aggravation of a TRD. The latter result is not so surprising because a correlation was found between the severity of retinopathy and TRD.

However, patients with macula threatening TRD were not examined in this study. A small study from Oshima et al., however, reported that patients with a ring shaped fibrovascular membrane may develop progressive TRD after anti-VEGF injection (Figs. 3.2, 3.3, 3.4 and 3.5) (Oshima et al. 2009). This occurred four days after injection. But all patients improved their vision despite the crunch (Arevalo et al. 2008).

Our treatment algorithm for non-macula threatening TRD is therefore an anti-VEGF treatment four weeks prior to vitrectomy. Our treatment algorithm for macula threatening TRD is anti-VEGF 3–5 days prior to vitrectomy (Fig. 3.6).

Our experience

Since 15 years we inject Avastin 4 weeks before surgery and had almost no problems with increased traction (crunch). In our opinion the anxiety about crunch is extremely over exaggerated. With consequent pretreatment, we could minimize the use of endodiathermy, minimize the amount of retinal tears, minimize the amount of postop hemorrhage and switch from silicone oil to gas tamponade. In a few cases, the TRD does contract a little but causes no harm. And you operate on a non-bleeding quiet eye and minimize the risk for postoperative PVR detachment. *Not once* did I regret the preoperative Avastin injection.

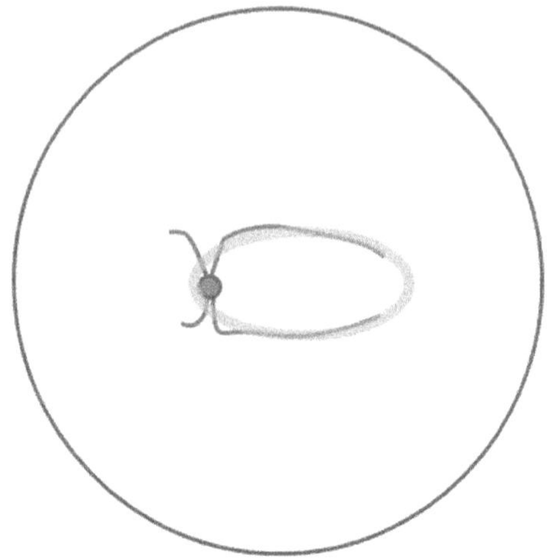

Fig. 3.2 A macula threatening and ring shaped TRD has an increased risk for aggravation of TRD after anti-VEGF injection. This eye we would treat 3–5 days before vitrectomy

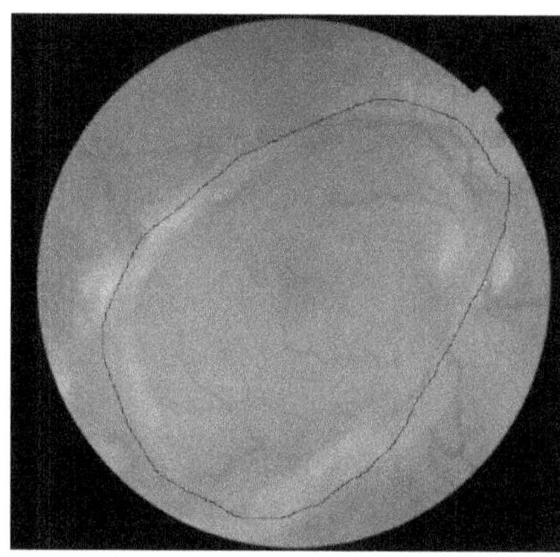

Fig. 3.3 A type 1 diabetic with a ring shaped TRD. This eye we would treat 3–5 days prior to surgery with anti-VEGF

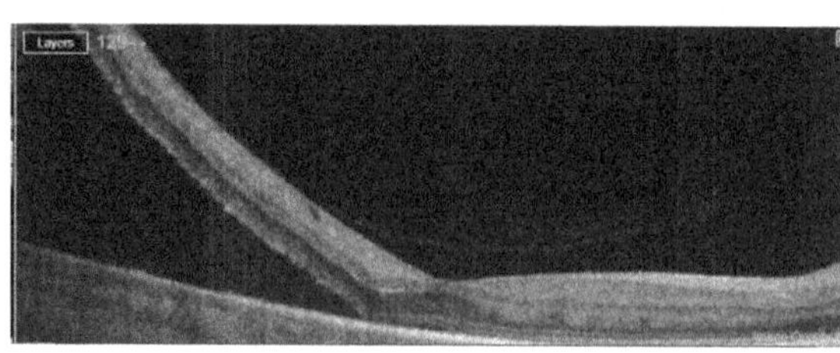

Fig. 3.4 The same patient as in Fig. 3.3. OCT, showing that the fovea is almost detached, VA = 1.0

Treatment planning of anti-VEGF injection

Another important aspect of preoperative anti-VEGF injection is the practical planning. If the patient has a long travel distance then a preoperative injection 3 days before surgery at our hospital is not possible. It could be done at the home hospital but the correct timing is very difficult and often too late or too early. In contrast,

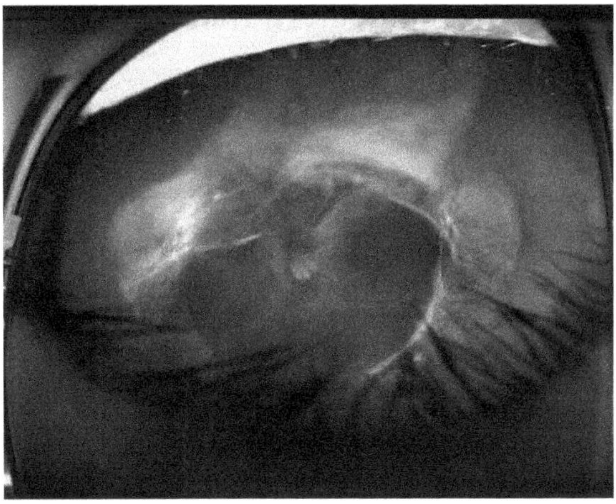

Fig. 3.5 This eye with ring shaped TRD has a high risk for aggravation of TRD after anti-VEGF injection. But would you operate this eye without an anti-VEGF pretreatment? We would not! The membrane does not threaten the macula but is very vascularized. We would treat this eye with anti-VEGF and schedule a vitrectomy in 4 weeks

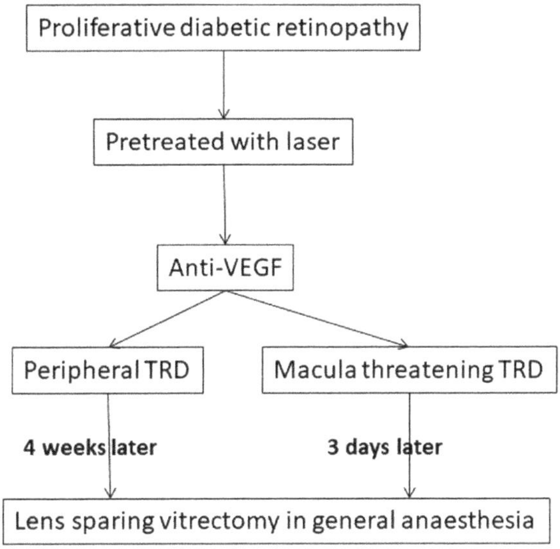

Fig. 3.6 Our treatment algorithm for eyes with TRD

a 4-week timing is easy for the home hospital or for the own hospital. An injection of 4 weeks ± 1 week is easy to plan, even an injection 4 weeks ± 2 weeks is acceptable. This is a very important reason why we chose such a long preoperative anti-VEGF injection time.

3.2 Complications of No Pretreatment

The complications of no pretreatment are as follows:

Difficult vitrectomy and long surgical time: A lack of pretreatment results in more retinal breaks, more intraoperative bleeding and more endodiathermy applications. During surgery you will experience preretinal, retinal and subretinal bleedings. These bleedings must be controlled and removed because they increase the risk of a PVR detachment. Depending on the severity of the retinopathy these bleedings are difficult and time consuming to control.

Increased risk for postoperative PVR detachment: During surgery you will experience preretinal, retinal and subretinal bleedings. These bleedings must be controlled and removed because they increase the risk of a PVR detachment. In case of a non-severe diabetic retinopathy, you may be able to cauterize them. But in case of a severe PDR, you will experience severe bleedings which are very difficult and time consuming to control. In addition, you will create huge retinal defects (Fig. 3.7). The surgical failure results in a functional failure.

Increased risk of postoperative hemorrhage: The risk for a postoperative hemorrhage is very high (Fig. 3.8) and increases the necessity for a silicone oil tamponade. Before we introduced pre and peroperative anti-VEGF treatment 1/3 of our patients had a postoperative hemorrhage. After we introduced a pre- and peroperative anti-VEGF treatment the incidence for postoperative hemorrhage reduced to almost zero. This observation is confirmed by recent studies (Smith and Steel 2015; Oshima et al. 2009).

Retinal damage: The retinal bleedings make the peeling difficult and increase the risk for retinal ruptures. Surgical trauma and severe hemorrhage may result in retinal damage. The consequence is a poor anatomical and functional outcome (Fig. 3.9).

Permanent silicone oil tamponade: A bad diabetic retinopathy without pretreatment results in a difficult vitrectomy, long surgical time and surgical complications. These complications necessitate a silicone oil tamponade which is in the most

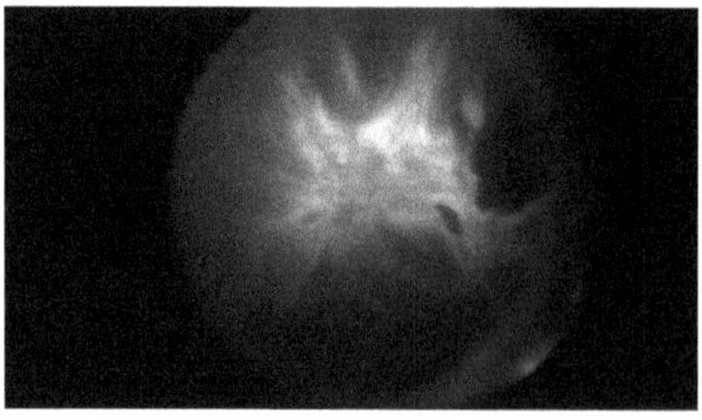

Fig. 3.7 Month after vitrectomy for diabetic retinopathy. Note the huge retinal defect. No anti-VEGF treatment was given before or during surgery

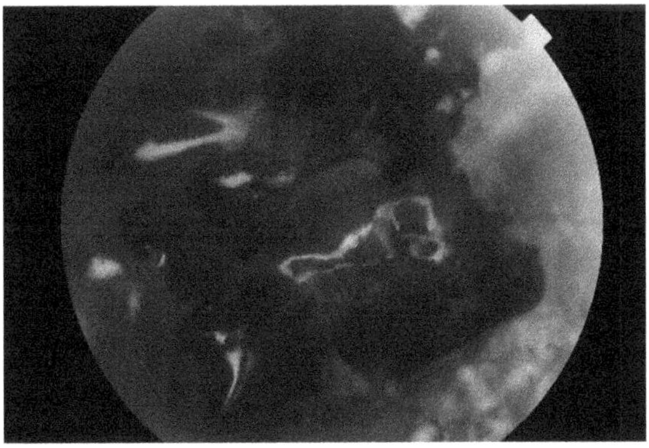

Fig. 3.8 Postoperative fundus. Extensive preretinal bleeding under silicone oil due to lack of pretreatment. Anti-VEGF was not injected preoperatively

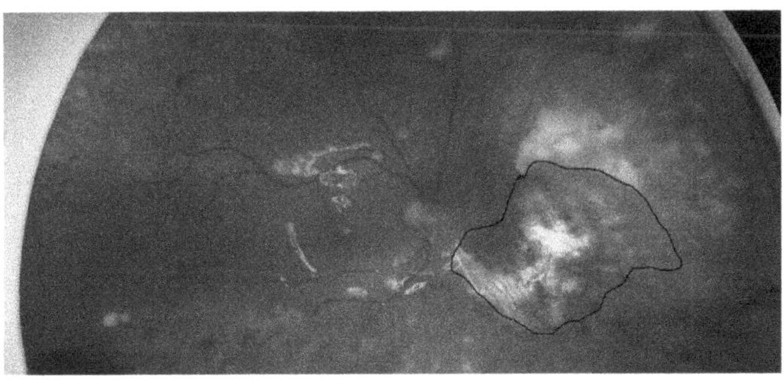

Fig. 3.9 Optos photograph, showing two years follow up after vitrectomy, peeling and silicone oil. Note huge retinal defect (black line) due to traumatic peeling. The white tissue at the defect is folded retina. Anti-VEGF was not injected prior surgery

cases permanent. A permanent silicone oil tamponade often causes IOP spikes resulting in a pale optic disc. Finally, the permanent silicone oil tamponade presses the posterior hyaloid with remaining membranes against the retina if not removed in the primary surgery.

A permanent silicone oil tamponade does not prevent a recurrence of proliferative membranes (Figs. 3.10 and 3.11). After 1 year of silicone oil tamponade, however, an additional vitrectomy is very difficult because a removal of the posterior hyaloid and membranes is very difficult and time consuming (Figs. 3.10 and 3.11).

An increased amount of reoperations: The risk for postoperative intravitreal hemorrhage (Figs. 3.8, 3.10 and 3.11) is high and necessitates a high number of reoperations such as lavage. A clinic that uses no anti-VEGF for diabetic vitrectomy has approximately 30% more reoperations compared to a clinic that uses

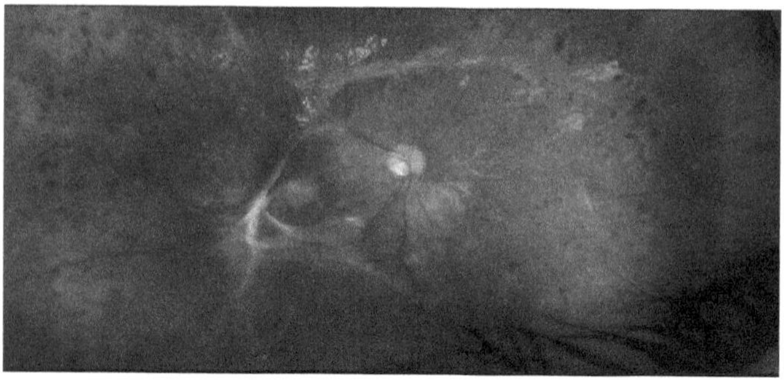

Fig. 3.10 Optos photograph, showing a 1-year follow up after vitrectomy with silicone oil for PDR. The silicone oil is since 1 year in the eye and presses all membranes and posterior hyaloid onto the underlying retina

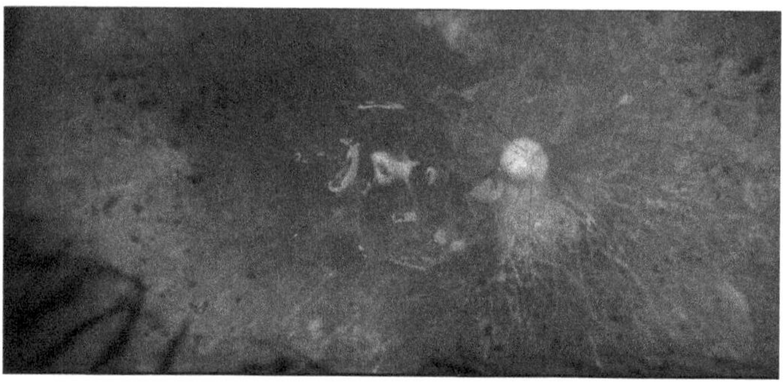

Fig. 3.11 After two vitrectomies with every two hours surgical time all membranes are removed. Optos photograph, showing that the posterior hyaloid was attached to the central pole and the membranes were extremely difficult to remove

consequently anti-VEGF for surgical cases (Oshima et al. 2009; Smith and Steel 2015). In case of a *bad* diabetic retinopathy, the number of possible reoperations is even higher. A vitrectomy with silicone oil tamponade necessitates also a second surgery for the removal of the oil.

Conclusion

The most common mistake in the eyes with TRD is an immediate surgery. In contrast, be hesitant with vitrectomy. Do not operate before the eye is adequately pretreated with anti-VEGF and laser. For vitreous hemorrhage, we recommend to wait 4 weeks. In case of a PDR with peripheral TRD, we wait 4 weeks but in case of a macula threatening TRD we inject 3 days prior to vitrectomy.

3.3 Sequential or Combined Phaco-Vitrectomy?

A vitrectomy in a pseudophakic eye is always easier than a vitrectomy in a phakic eye. There are only two indications for a combined phaco/vitrectomy: A rhegmatogenous retinal detachment and trauma surgery. Otherwise, a phacoemulsification can be performed in the first step and then a vitrectomy can be done in the second step. A stepwise approach reduces the peroperative complications, facilitates the removal of anterior vitreous and removes the necessity of a delayed and difficult cataract surgery. Diabetic patients have an impaired wound healing. A combined approach increases inflammation in an already inflamed and proliferative eye. A sequential (two-step) phaco-vitrectomy results in a rapid visual acuity recovery. Why? Because two-step phaco-vitrectomy minimizes postoperative vitreous hemorrhage which is significantly more frequent after combined phaco-vitrectomy (Rivas-Aguiño et al. 2009).

Conclusion: No, no combined phaco/vitrectomy. A combined phaco/vitrectomy causes inflammation and increased postoperative vitreous hemorrhage. Perform first a phaco and IOL implantation combined with an anti-VEGF injection and a few weeks later (I prefer 4 weeks) a safe vitrectomy can be performed.

3.4 Immediate Vitrectomy? Yes or No?

There is no necessity for an immediate vitrectomy for diabetic vitrectomy. The retinal changes in diabetic retinopathy are chronic and progress slowly. An eye with partial vitreous hemorrhage and TRD does not require an immediate vitrectomy. The main impetus for an immediate vitrectomy is a VR surgeon who is excited to perform a challenging surgery but this is not in the best interest of the eye. These difficult eyes which have chronic changes require a good treatment planning which includes a delayed vitrectomy. Reduce the proliferative and inflammatory activity until you have a quiet retinopathy. Then the TRD can be removed safely without causing complications or even a failure.

Conclusion: No, no immediate vitrectomy. Instead, a *delayed* vitrectomy is required. Pretreat the eye first with anti-VEGF and laser. If you plan a lens removal then choose a two-step approach.

The following video shows two advanced diabetic cases: Chapter 3: Two extreme cases of diabetic retinopathy.

3.5 Summary

Avastin has a positive effect in 100% of patients and a negative effect in 3,5% (Arevalo et al. 2019). Is it advisable not to inject Avastin in these 3,5% of patients? No. Why? Because all patients improved vision despite crunch. In addition, you lose the positive effect of Avastin. Which positive effect? Preoperative Avastin reduces the severity of diabetic retinopathy (Bressler et al. 2020) resulting in a less complicated vitrectomy. This implies less intraoperative bleeding, less endodiathermy, less iatrogenic ruptures, less silicone oil tamponade and last but not least less surgical failures.

References

Arevalo JF, Maia M, Flynn HW Jr, et al. Tractional retinal detachment following intravitreal bevacizumab (Avastin) in patients with severe proliferative diabetic retinopathy. Br J Ophthalmol. 2008;92(2):213–6.

Arevalo JF, Lasave AF, Kozak I, Al Rashaed S, Al Kahtani E, Maia M, Farah ME, Cutolo C, Brito M, Osorio C, Navarro P, Wu L, Berrocal MH, Morales-Canton V, Serrano MA, Graue-Wiechers F, Sabrosa NA, Alezzandrini AA, Gallego-Pinazo R. Pan-American Collaborative Retina Study (PACORES) Group. Preoperative Bevacizumab for tractional retinal detachment in proliferative diabetic retinopathy: a prospective randomized clinical trial. Am J Ophthalmol. 2019; 207:279–287. https://doi.org/10.1016/j.ajo.2019.05.007. Epub 2019 May 13. PMID: 31095954.

Bressler NM, Beaulieu WT, Bressler SB, Glassman AR, Melia BM, Jampol LM, Jhaveri CD, Salehi-Had H, Velez G, Sun JK; DRCR Retina Network. Anti-vascular endothelial growth factor therapy and risk of traction retinal detachment in eyes with proliferative diabetic retinopathy: pooled analysis of five DRCR retina network randomized clinical trials. Retina. 2020; 40(6):1021–1028.

Oshima Y, Shima C, Wakabayashi T, Kusaka S, Shiraga F, Ohji M, Tano Y. Microincision vitrectomy surgery and intravitreal bevacizumab as a surgical adjunct to treat diabetic traction retinal detachment. Ophthalmology. 2009;116(5):927–38.

Rivas-Aguiño P, García-Amaris RA, Berrocal MH, Sánchez JG, Rivas A, Arévalo JF. Vitrectomía pars plana, facoemulsificación e implante de lente intraocular para el manejo de catarata y retinopatía diabética proliferativa: comparación de técnica quirúrgica combinada versus en dos tiempos [Pars plana vitrectomy, phacoemulsification and intraocular lens implantation for the management of cataract and proliferative diabetic retinopathy: comparison of a combined versus two-step surgical approach]. Arch Soc Esp Oftalmol. 2009; 84(1):31–8. Spanish. https://doi.org/10.4321/s0365-66912009000100005. PMID: 19173136.

Smith JM, Steel DH. Anti-vascular endothelial growth factor for prevention of postoperative vitreous cavity haemorrhage after vitrectomy for proliferative diabetic retinopathy. Cochrane Database Syst Rev. 2015; 2015(8):CD008214.

Part II

Treatment Planning

4 Surgical Scenarios

There are three typical main scenarios for diabetic vitrectomy (Diabetic Retinopathy Research Group 1981). The *first* main scenario is an old patient (60–80 y/o) with type 2 diabetes. A vitreous hemorrhage is present and the posterior vitreous is *detached* (Fig. 4.1). A scatter laser treatment has been performed. A tractional retinal detachment (TRD) is not present. This eye may be phakic or pseudophakic. This is surgically an easy diabetic vitrectomy.

The *second* main scenario is a middle aged (40–60 y/o) patient with type 1 or 2 diabetes. A vitreous hemorrhage is present. There is no view to the fundus. Some scatter laser has been performed. A TRD is present and the posterior vitreous is attached only at a few places (Fig. 4.2). The eye is usually phakic. This is a presumed easy but in reality, a difficult diabetic vitrectomy.

The *third* main scenario is a young patient (20–40 y/o) with insulin dependent diabetes (type 1 diabetes). There is a good view to fundus but a mild vitreous hemorrhage may be present. A tractional retinal detachment (Fig. 4.3) is present where the posterior vitreous is *attached* at many places. In most cases due to poor compliance, no PRP has been performed. The eye has a natural lens. This is surgically a difficult diabetic vitrectomy.

A thorough pre-surgical examination of the diabetic fundus is important but can be misleading. A preoperatively simple case may become intraoperatively very difficult. Why? Not all cases have fibrovascular membranes indicating severe retinopathy. Essential for diabetic surgery is the status of the posterior hyaloid. Is a posterior vitreous detachment (PVD) present or not? The more complete the PVD the better, because the attached posterior vitreous causes tractions on the retina. Remark: All diabetic eyes without PVD are surgically difficult and demanding regarding surgery and the postoperative course.

U. Spandau and Z. Tomic, *Small-Gauge Vitrectomy for Diabetic Retinopathy*,
https://doi.org/10.1007/978-3-031-26204-3_4

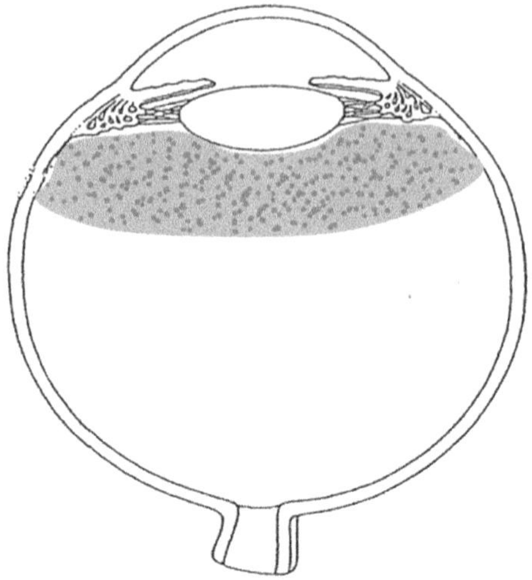

Fig. 4.1 First main scenario: A completely detached posterior hyaloid typically associated with vitreous hemorrhage. There are no fibrovascular membranes at the posterior pole. This is an easy diabetic vitrectomy

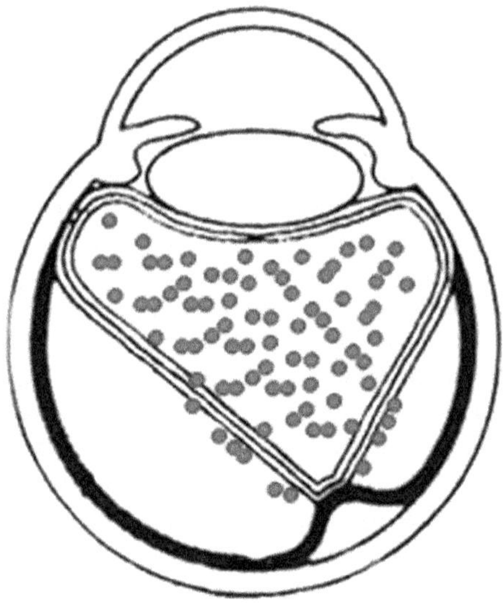

Fig. 4.2 Second main scenario: Drawing of a PDR with TRD. A vitreous hemorrhage is present. The posterior hyaloid is attached causing a few focal detachments. This is a difficult diabetic vitrectomy

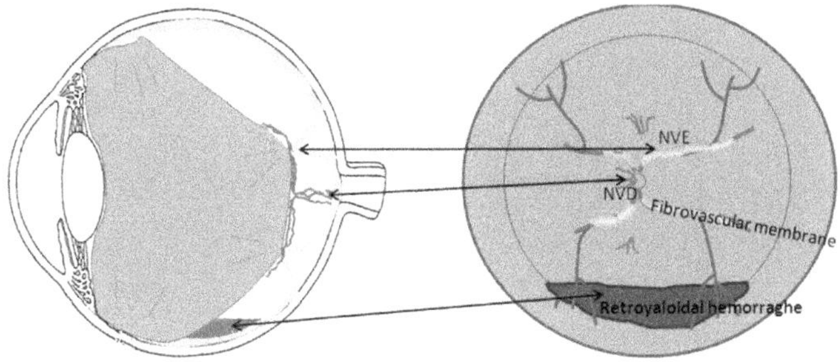

Fig. 4.3 Third main scenario: Drawing of a severe PDR with TRD. The posterior hyaloid is attached at several places causing focal detachments. This is a difficult diabetic vitrectomy

Reference

Diabetic Retinopathy Research Group. Invest Ophthalmol Vis Sci. 1981; 21:210

Indication and Aim of Vitrectomy of a Diabetic Eye

5

5.1 Indication and Aim of Vitrectomy

The main indications for a diabetic vitrectomy are (1) To clear the media in order to enable us to do laser photocoagulation (2) To release the traction causing visual loss or threatening to cause so and (3) To arrest the process of progressive PDR in spite of an adequate PRP, e.g., persistent neovascularization of iris.

The aim of diabetic vitrectomy is ZERO failure. Zero failure means no PVR detachment after vitrectomy for PDR. This aim is achievable if you follow the guidelines of this book. In my University clinic, we have no PVR detachments after diabetic vitrectomy because we follow these guidelines. And in Sweden, we have very advanced tractional diabetic retinopathies.

The main steps of vitrectomy for diabetic retinopathy are the removal of posterior vitreous and laser photocoagulation. The removal of posterior vitreous may be very difficult due to strong adhesions between retina and posterior hyaloid. Laser photocoagulation is the most essential treatment modality for an ischemic retinopathy because it results in a final regression of retinal proliferations and finally in an inactive PDR (Fig. 5.1).

The most difficult step of vitrectomy is the induction of posterior vitreous detachment. Why? The posterior hyaloid is firmly adherent to the retina in many advanced PDR patients. These adhesions have to be dissected and delaminated with a blunt instrument and intravitreal scissors (posterior hyaloid separation). If you simply perform a central PVD with the vitreous cutter you may cause retinal tears and damage the blood vessels because of the strong pull of inducing PVD causing a rip in retina due to strong attachments (Fig. 5.2).

With diabetes, wounds tend to heal more slowly and get infected easily and a diabetic eye has an increased vascular and inflammatory activity. Therefore, a stepwise treatment planning is the key to success. This means that we do a sequential and not a combined phaco/vitrectomy. We start with a phacoemulsification (plus intravitreal Avastin) and continue 4 weeks later with vitrectomy. The

U. Spandau and Z. Tomic, *Small-Gauge Vitrectomy for Diabetic Retinopathy*,
https://doi.org/10.1007/978-3-031-26204-3_5

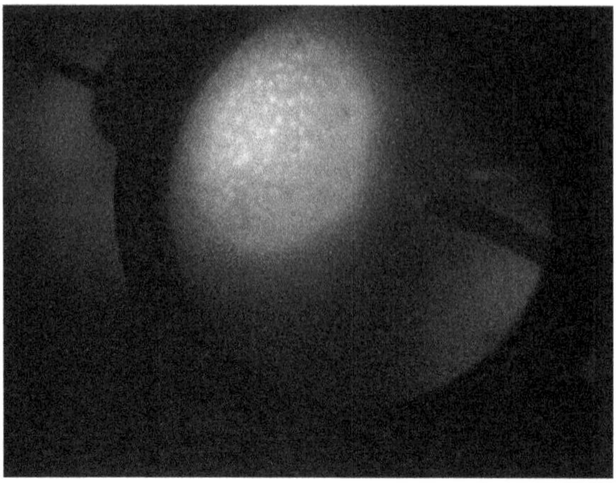

Fig. 5.1 Perform a PRP up to the ora serrata

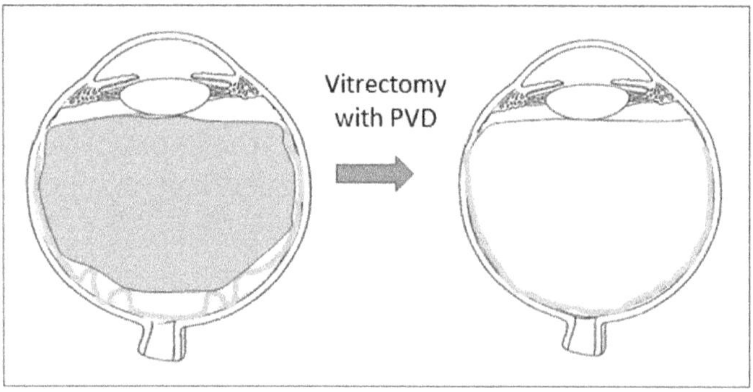

Fig. 5.2 The left eye shows the status of posterior hyaloid and retina before vitrectomy. The right eye shows a removed vitreous including posterior hyaloid and an attached retina

stepwise approach reduces surgical trauma and the use of anti-VEGF reduces the vascular activity before and prepares the eye for the delayed vitrectomy. With anti-VEGF treatment, the vascular component decreases and a more fibrotic component remains. In addition, the risk for postoperative vitreous hemorrhage is very much reduced.

5.2 Do Not Operate on These Patients

Be careful what eyes you choose to operate. In case of a surgical failure, you may regret your choice. Be cautious with the following pathologies:

Optic atrophy: Eyes with optic atrophy and no light perception should not be operated.

Burnt out PDR: Eyes with burnt out PDR and no light perception should not be operated.

Neovascular glaucoma: Eyes with neovascularization of the iris and no light perception should not be operated. If, however, this eye becomes painful due to high intraocular pressure then the eye should be operated with the aim of eye preservation. Eyes with neovascular glaucoma and useful vision must be operated with the aim of vision preservation. We have a simple and novel treatment planning and surgical technique for this pathology. See chapter "Neovascular glaucoma".

Summary:

The aim of vitrectomy is the clearing of a vitreous hemorrhage, induction of posterior vitreous detachment with removal of membranes and a scatter laser photocoagulation to achieve an inactive PDR. An easy case at the slit lamp may become a difficult case on the surgical table. The most common cause for failure of vitrectomy for proliferative diabetic retinopathy is to operate on a naive eye (untreated). Operate instead only an eye that has been treated prior vitrectomy with scatter laser and anti-VEGF.

Treatment Planning

6

6.1 Preoperative Intravitreal Anti-VEGF and Sequential Phaco/Vitrectomy

The treatment planning of the diabetic eye is essential for surgical success. What is the right timing for a vitrectomy? Many VR surgeons perform an immediate vitrectomy. We avoid an immediate vitrectomy because the risk for surgical failure is high. We recommend instead an immediate treatment with anti-VEGF and laser if possible and a delayed vitrectomy. If the eye is not pretreated with PRP or anti-VEGF injections and the diabetes is poorly controlled, then the vitrectomy gets very difficult. The best timing for a vitrectomy is when the fibrovascular membranes are dry and avascular. The main rule is not to perform a vitrectomy in an untreated active PDR eye. Pretreat the eye first with anti-VEGF and PRP if possible, keep a tight follow-up until the retinopathy is quiet and then schedule surgery.

For surgery of diabetic eyes, we favour a stepwise procedure, i.e., we operate in several sessions depending on the severity of the PDR. Why a stepwise procedure? Diabetes affects wound healing. A severe diabetic retinopathy requires a long traumatic surgery. The surgical trauma causes inflammation and aggravates the diabetic retinopathy, resulting in a vicious cycle. The difficulty of the vitrectomy depends on the severity of the PDR.

Remark: The treatment planning is, however, determined by local factors such as reimbursement of the surgery or the travel distance to the hospital. If the costs of the surgery are covered by the national health system and the patient lives close by then you, as a surgeon, have much more freedom for treatment planning (Author US in Sweden). If the travel distance is long then the pretreatment must be done at the home clinic. We ask the home clinic to perform an anti-VEGF injection and schedule a vitrectomy one month later (Author ZT in Serbia).

U. Spandau and Z. Tomic, *Small-Gauge Vitrectomy for Diabetic Retinopathy*,
https://doi.org/10.1007/978-3-031-26204-3_6

6.2 Surgery of Easy Diabetic Vitrectomy

The typical patient is a 75 y/o patient with type II diabetes. For 3 months a vitreous hemorrhage is present with no tendency of resorption. A complete PVD is present and the eye is scatter laser treated (Fig. 6.1).

Our treatment algorithm is a sequential phaco/vitrectomy.

We start with a phacoemulsification plus anti-VEGF injection (Fig. 6.2). Four weeks later we schedule a vitrectomy. The vitreous hemorrhage is removed, a fill in PRP performed, anti-VEGF injected and finalized with an air/gas tamponade.

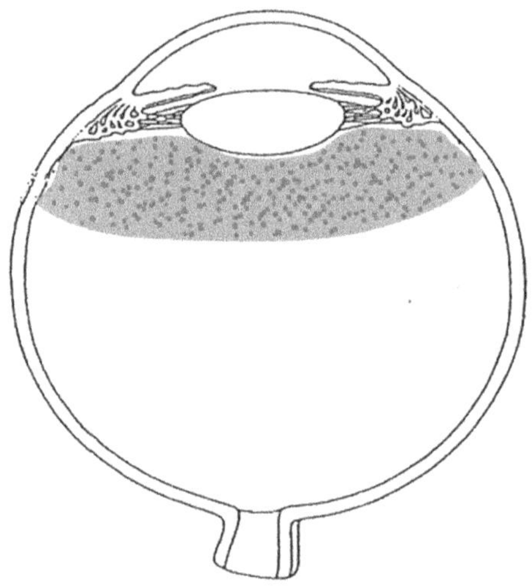

Fig. 6.1 A diabetic retinopathy with vitreous hemorrhage. Note that a complete PVD is present. Fibrovascular membranes are usually not present because the posterior hyaloid is detached. The usual age is >60 years. We perform always a two-step phacoemulsification/vitrectomy

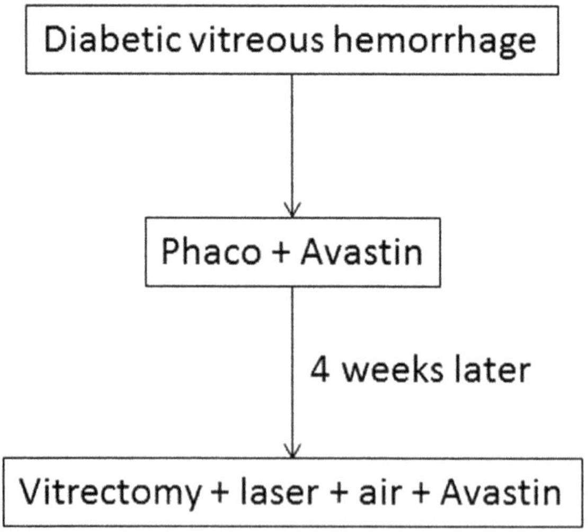

Fig. 6.2 Our treatment planning algorithm for surgically easy PDR. Note the sequential phaco/vitrectomy

We prefer this stepwise procedure because diabetic eyes have a high tendency for inflammatory reaction. Four weeks after phacoemulsification the anterior segment is quiet and no iris rubeosis or posterior synechiae develop. The anti-VEGF injection stops the active vitreous bleeding and the risk for postoperative vitreous hemorrhage is extremely reduced. In addition, the anti-VEGF treatment results in a regression of the grade of diabetic retinopathy.

Surgical pearls

Vitreous hemorrhage: A diabetic eye with vitreous hemorrhage requires PRP. A PRP is, however, not possible. Inject intravitreal 0.1 ml Avastin and wait approximately 4 weeks. If there is no improvement after 4 weeks we schedule a vitrectomy. If the vitreous has cleared we perform a PRP according to the extent of the retinal ischemia. Several patients do not require a vitrectomy in the end. Many vitrectomies can be avoided if the patients are properly pretreated with laser and anti-VEGF.

6.3 (Surgical) Difficult Diabetic Vitrectomy Case, Where Retina Already Pretreated with Scatter Laser

A typical case is a middle-aged patient with type 1 or 2 diabetes. The posterior vitreous is attached at a few places and fibrovascular membranes are present (Fig. 6.3). The hyaloid is partially detached in the periphery but the nasal posterior hyaloid is often attached. Usually, these eyes are partially treated with scatter laser. The aim of surgery is to induce a PVD and remove the posterior hyaloid together with the fibrovascular membranes.

We operate in two sessions. Our treatment planning is depicted in Fig. 6.4. First, we inject anti-VEGF. In case of a peripheral TRD, we schedule a vitrectomy four

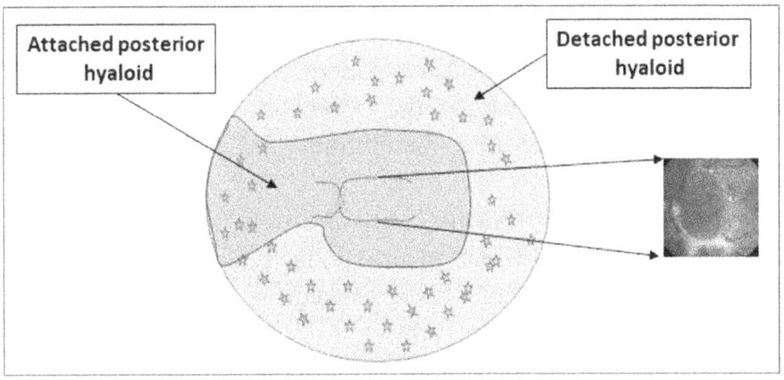

Fig. 6.3 Illustration of a PDR with TRD and the anatomy of the posterior vitreous. A PRP has been performed. The posterior hyaloid is attached in the posterior pole and partially detached in the superior, temporal and inferior periphery; the nasal posterior hyaloid is often attached

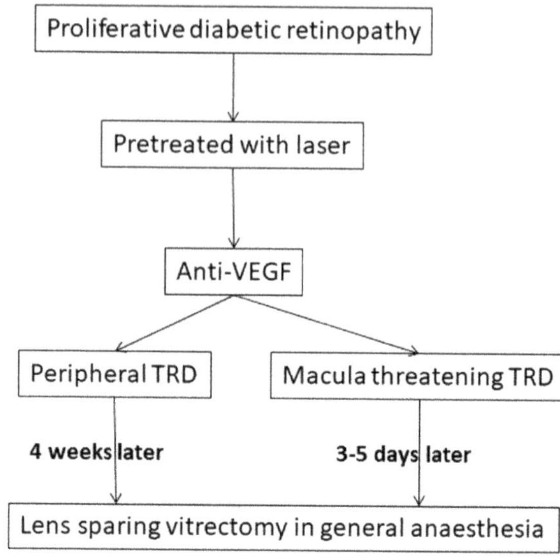

Fig. 6.4 Flow chart of our treatment planning of PDR. The retina is already treated with scatter laser. Note the different timing for macula threatening and peripheral TRD

weeks later but in case of a macula threatening, we schedule a vitrectomy after 3–5 days. Remark: These patients are usually operated in general anaesthesia.

Caution: The presurgical examination of a diabetic fundus can be misleading. A preoperatively simple case may become intraoperatively very difficult. The eye may have hidden vitreoretinal adhesions and extensive bleeding may occur after induction of PVD. **Remember:** A proliferative diabetic eye with attached posterior vitreous is always a difficult surgical case.

6.4 (Surgical) Difficult Diabetic Vitrectomy Case NOT Pretreated with Scatter Laser

A typical case is a young type I diabetic patient with bad compliance. The eye is not treated with PRP or anti-VEGF, the posterior vitreous is attached at many places, and extensive fibrovascular membranes and tractional detachments are present.

We perform a three-step procedure. See the treatment algorithm in Fig. 6.5. We start with an immediate Avastin injection and schedule a LIO laser treatment in general anaesthesia. Four weeks later we plan an additional laser treatment if media clears up or schedule a vitrectomy.

What is the rationale of this treatment planning? Never operate in an angry PDR, make it quiescent before surgery. Do not operate an eye with advanced diabetic retinopathy, which is not pretreated with anti-VEGF or PRP. If the retina is attached, then perform a PRP and inject anti-VEGF medication. If the retina is partially detached, then laser treat the attached retina. These advanced eyes

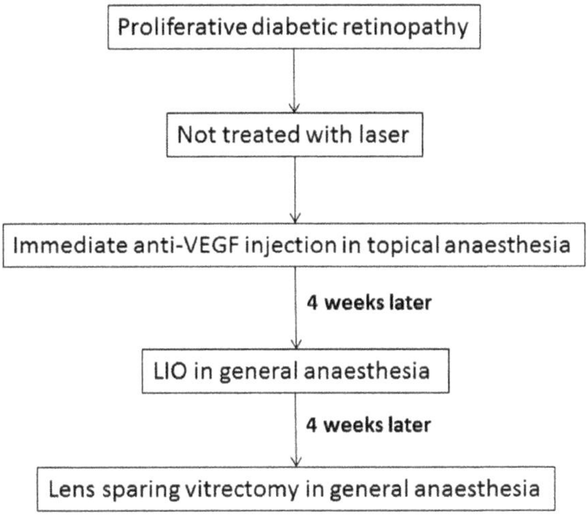

Fig. 6.5 Our treatment planning for an advanced diabetic retinopathy. We employ a three-step treatment algorithm; first anti-VEGF, then PRP and in a third step, vitrectomy

are like a VEGF forest fire. A vitrectomy will add extra fuel to the fire. Extinguish the fire with PRP and anti-VEGF and perform a vitrectomy at a later time point when the VEGF load is low and PDR is inactive. At the time of vitrectomy, the fibrovascular membranes should be white and dry i.e., avascular (fibrous component dominating). Now the risk for a peroperative bleeding is minimal (Fig. 6.6).

Caution: In case of a metabolically unstable and young type I diabetic, we wait with the vitrectomy as long as possible. We treat the eye with anti-VEGF and

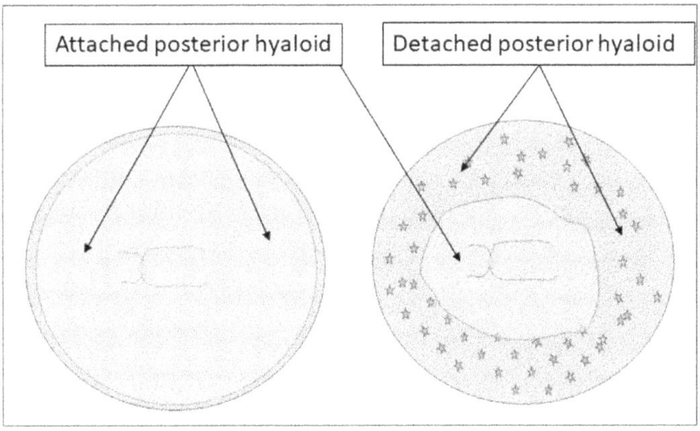

Fig. 6.6 The fundus on the left shows a completely attached posterior hyaloid in a young diabetic. No scatter laser has been done. The fundus on the right side shows the same eye after scatter laser. The scatter laser has induced a peripheral PVD. The posterior hyaloid is still attached at the posterior pole together with fibrovascular membranes. The vitrectomy is much easier now

PRP and wait. If a focal detachment involves the macula you have to perform a vitrectomy. If a focal detachment in the nasal quadrant remains stable then wait. These eyes must be treated like raw eggs.

Summary:

TRD secondary to diabetes is the most difficult and challenging vitrectomy. Many VR surgeons fail operating these eyes. The biggest mistake is an immediate surgery. Instead start with an immediate treatment with laser and anti-VEGF and schedule a delayed vitrectomy. In case of an easy diabetic vitrectomy start with phacoemulsification and anti-VEGF injection and schedule a vitrectomy four weeks later. In case of a presumed difficult diabetic vitrectomy inject first anti-VEGF. If possible perform then a PRP. Then schedule a vitrectomy 4 weeks later unless a macula threatening membrane is present- in the latter case, we schedule vitrectomy after 3–5 days after anti-VEGF injection.

Part III

General Aspects and Surgical Techniques About Anti-VEGF, Laser Photocoagulation and Vitrectomy for Diabetic Retinopathy

General Aspects and Surgical Techniques About Anti-VEGF, Laser Photocoagulation and Vitrectomy for Diabetic Retinopathy

7

7.1 Three Weapons Against Diabetic Retinopathy

We have three weapons against proliferative diabetic retinopathy.

(1) Laser photocoagulation
(2) Anti-VEGF injections
(3) Vitrectomy

The most important weapon is laser photocoagulation because it results in a permanent cure of this otherwise blinding disease. The famous double-blind ETRDS study examined the effect of laser photocoagulation in eyes with PDR (1991). The eyes were randomized in laser treatment and no laser treatment. The results revealed a high efficacy of laser photocoagulation in the treated eyes and a high risk for severe visual acuity decrease in the non-treated eyes. Laser is the most important treatment for PDR. This notion is confirmed by an interesting study which treated patients with anti-VEGF or laser photocoagulation for PDR (Obeid et al. 2019). After a delayed follow-up of more than 1 year (due to loss of follow up of patients), eyes with laser treatment did well and had a good anatomical and functional outcome. In contrast, eyes with anti-VEGF treatment had a significantly greater incidence of neovascularization of the iris and poor functional outcome. This study demonstrates that laser has a sustaining long effect but the effect of anti-VEGF is short and will need frequent dosing.

Since 2003 we have a second weapon against diabetic retinopathy which pushed laser away from its throne. The anti-VEGF treatment proved to be so effective against PDR that it has replaced laser photocoagulation as first line treatment in the USA (2). Anti-VEGF does not cause visual field defects, photopsias, transient loss of accommodation and macular edema as is the case for laser photocoagulation. In 43% of patients, PDR did not reoccur after termination of anti-VEGF treatment (Sun et al. 2019). But in 30% of patients, anti-VEGF treatment has to be repeated

U. Spandau and Z. Tomic, *Small-Gauge Vitrectomy for Diabetic Retinopathy*,
https://doi.org/10.1007/978-3-031-26204-3_7

continuously resulting in an increased risk for endophthalmitis and systemic side effects. Until this problem is solved, laser photocoagulation will continue to be an essential treatment modality for diabetic retinopathy.

If a nationwide screening program exists, then anti-VEGF and laser photocoagulation are sufficient to treat diabetic retinopathy. An efficient screening program and laser photocoagulation are the most cost-effective treatment modalities against diabetic retinopathy because a costly vitrectomy can be avoided. For a nationwide treatment of diabetic retinopathy, the use of laser photocoagulation machines are far more effective than vitrectomy machines.

But even an effective screening program and a surplus of laser machines cannot avoid that some patients have a lack of compliance and fall through the screening net.

The typical patient in our country is a 35-year-old female patient with type 1 diabetes and bilateral PDR. One eye has very poor vision and the fellow eye has recently experienced a visual acuity decrease. Both eyes have never been treated with laser photocoagulation or anti-VEGF. The patient missed all calls for screening. The first thing we do in these patients is to treat them immediately with a bilateral anti-VEGF injection. An anti-VEGF injection wins time for further planning. We then perform a bilateral LIO (laser indirect ophthalmoscopy) combined with a second anti-VEGF injection. The vitrectomy is scheduled 4 weeks later. Now the risk for intraoperative bleeding is very low and the laser photocoagulation induced a partial PVD, facilitating a removal of the central hyaloid during vitrectomy. LIO and vitrectomy are planned in general anaesthesia because the surgery is difficult and the patients have a poor compliance.

7.2 Preoperative Anti-VEGF-Treatment

Anti-VEGF agents are an essential part in the armamentarium of a retinal surgeon to treat diabetic retinopathy. They can be used pre-, intra and postoperatively. The most important time to inject is preoperatively. If you plan to operate an active PDR then inject anti-VEGF. We usually inject 1–4 weeks before vitrectomy. The proliferative vessels are regressed when you perform vitrectomy and the bleeding is significantly reduced during surgery.

Another excellent indication for anti-VEGF treatment is a vitreous hemorrhage of diabetic origin. A laser treatment is not possible due to media opacity. But an anti-VEGF injection treats the underlying pathology and stops the vitreous bleeding making the subsequent vitrectomy easy. In addition, the risk of postoperative hemorrhage is reduced.

Is anti-VEGF indicated in tractional detachment? We inject anti-VEGF agents even in eyes with tractional detachment and did not observe progression of a tractional detachment. All anti-VEGF agents on the market (Lucentis®, Eylea®, Avastin®) can be used for treatment.

Use **caution** regarding the timing of phaco and anti-VEGF treatment. The effect of Avastin lasts 6 weeks. After 4–6 weeks, a laser treatment with/without vitrectomy should be scheduled. Repeat alternatively an anti-VEGF injection. Otherwise, the PDR will reoccur after 2–3 months.

7.3 Laser Treatment: Laser Indirect Ophthalmoscopy (LIO) and Endolaser

In case of not-advanced PDR, we use slit lamp laser. The laser energy is absorbed by melanin in RPE and choroid and also by haemoglobin in blood. The heat generated by the laser also diffuses to the outer retina and photoreceptors. The nerve fibre layer and the inner retina are not affected in case of a pascal photo coagulator due to less thermal diffusion (30 ms duration burns) (Fig. 7.1). However, with a double frequency Nd Yag or Argon laser there is thermal diffusion from RPE and choroid leading to damage of the ganglion cell layer and inner retina. This destruction of the outer retina results in chorioretinal scars through which oxygen flows from the choroid to inner retina. Furthermore the destruction of ischemic tissue in the retina causes reduction of the VEGF load leading to improvement of ischemia and regression of the retinal proliferations.

If a laser treatment at the slit lamp is not possible because of a lack of compliance or disability, it is possible to perform a laser treatment with a binocular head ophthalmoscope called LIO (Laser indirect ophthalmoscope), (Fig. 7.2). A complete scatter laser of all four quadrants can be performed within one session. General anaesthesia is recommended. A LIO treatment is very helpful in young diabetic type I patients with low compliance. You can place approximately 1200–1800 laser spots in each eye and add an anti-VEGF injection to prevent a macular edema. For details see Sect. 11.1 Laser indirect photocoagulation of the retina".

Surgical pearls

Effect of Laser: Laser treatment reduces the retinal proliferation AND induces often a partial PVD. A vitrectomy is much easier in an eye with partial PVD.

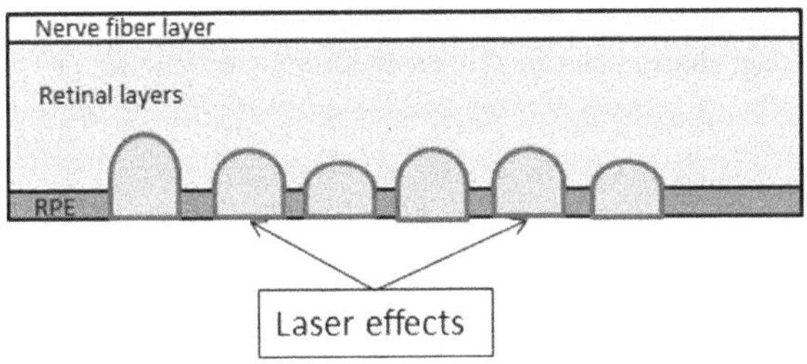

Fig. 7.1 Effects of laser burns in the retina with pascal laser. The nerve fibre layer is not affected because the thermal diffusion is low with a 30 ms spot but with a conventional laser, a 100 ms spot causes a 200μ thermal diffusion causing some collateral damage to the inner retina

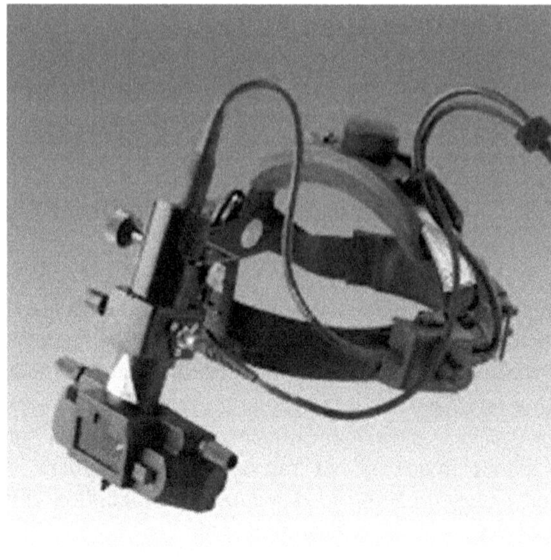

Fig. 7.2 Headset and cable for laser indirect ophthalmoscope (Ellex, Australia). The cable is connected to a laser device

Surgical pearls

LIO treatment: Young type 1 diabetics and generally diabetic patients with discomfort for slit lamp laser treatment are good candidates for LIO treatment. Why? With LIO you can treat the complete retina. LIO is however painful and is best performed in general anaesthesia but is also possible in retrobulbar anaesthesia. You can perform a dense PRP up to the ora serrata within one session in both eyes. We add anti-VEGF to prevent a macular edema.

7.4 Cryopexy

An effective alternative to laser is cryopexy. We use cryopexy always for neovascular glaucoma because laser photocoagulation does not give the desired effect. The cryopexy effects destroy the choroid and retina whereas laser only destroys the outer retina. But in case of PDR, we do not use cryopexy because it induces more PVR reaction than laser. In our experience, the risk for a PVR detachment is increased after cryopexy treatment (in eyes with PDR but not in eyes with neovascular glaucoma).

7.5 Don't Forget the Fellow Eye

Most patients with PDR have a bilateral involvement and usually one eye is more affected than the other. During the time when you treat the first eye do not forget the fellow eye. This eye also needs a treatment, maybe only a laser photocoagulation or an anti-VEGF injection. We experienced many times that the fellow eye deteriorated and lost function because all the effort and time was placed on the poor eye. The reason for this is the long treatment and healing time of one eye. This may take 3–6 months and this is a long time for an active PDR.

7.6 Two-Step Phaco/Vitrectomy: Phaco + Anti-VEGF-Treatment

In all eyes under 50 years of age, we perform a lens-sparing vitrectomy. In all eyes over 50 years, we usually perform first a combined phaco and intravitreal anti-VEGF injection and 4 weeks later the vitrectomy. What is the rationale of this procedure? A vitrectomy in a pseudophakic eye is less traumatic than a combined phaco/vitrectomy and minimises postoperative vitreous hemorrhage. This may not be so relevant in a macular pucker surgery, but it is of utmost importance in an inflamed and vascular active pathology such as diabetic retinopathy. Diabetes delays the healing process. A cataract surgery increases significantly the activity of a proliferative diabetic retinopathy. An eye with a severe NPDR may develop a rubeotic iris after cataract surgery. To counteract the surgical trauma and inflammation of phacoemulsification, we perform an intravitreal anti-VEGF injection at the same time point. Furthermore, a diabetic vitrectomy is a planned surgery compared to an urgent surgery like a retinal detachment surgery. There is, therefore, no need for a combined surgery.

If you perform phacoemulsification without anti-VEGF, then you risk increasing the activity of the diabetic retinopathy. We never experienced a worsening of the diabetic retinopathy after phaco + Avastin; in contrast, the diabetic retinopathy improved in all cases. In some cases, the vitreous hemorrhage improves and a subsequent vitrectomy becomes unnecessary.

Remark to lensectomy: Perform phacoemulsification through cornea and place always an IOL into the bag. Avoid lensectomy from pars plana. Why? First of all, a lensectomy is not necessary. Secondly, a lensectomy implies a traumatic surgery which aggravates the diabetic retinopathy and results in the removal of lens capsule and aphakia. An aphakic eye without lens capsule and IOL has many disadvantages regarding vision and surgery. Regarding vision: The eye is aphakic and amblyopic. The patient needs a contact lens. Regarding surgery: The absent lens capsule cannot serve as a barrier for anterior and posterior segments and silicone oil or gas can prolapse into the anterior chamber. The risk for secondary glaucoma is increased. And last but not least, a secondary IOL implantation has to be performed.

7.7 Diabetic Vitrectomy

All gauges from 23 to 27G can be used for diabetic retinopathy. The most common gauge for diabetic retinopathy today is 25G. The reason is that all required instruments are available for 25-gauge. The best vitreous cutter for diabetic retinopathy, however, is the 27G vitreous cutter because the opening is very close to the cutter tip and you can easily cut tractional membranes. A good alternative is the bevelled 25G cutter from Alcon. This feature allows a dissection and cutting of tractional membranes.

25G vitrectomy: 25G is a good option for severe cases. For membrane dissection, we use a knob spatula (Eye Tech, UK) or a silicone tip flute needle and straight scissors (Eye Tech, UK).

27G vitrectomy: We use 27G for severe and easy cases (Fig. 7.3). The main reason for using 27G is the superior design of the vitreous cutter which allows a dissection of membranes (Fig. 7.4). If the peeling gets difficult, we change to a hybrid system and use 25G straight scissors. For example, 27G 3-port vitrectomy with chandelier illumination started: If a special instrument is required intraoperatively, which is only available in 25G, then you remove one 27G trocar and insert instead one 25G trocar, i.e., "hybrid system". Some instruments such as knob spatula and straight scissors are only available in 25G. Good alternatives are the curved scissors from DORC in 27G.

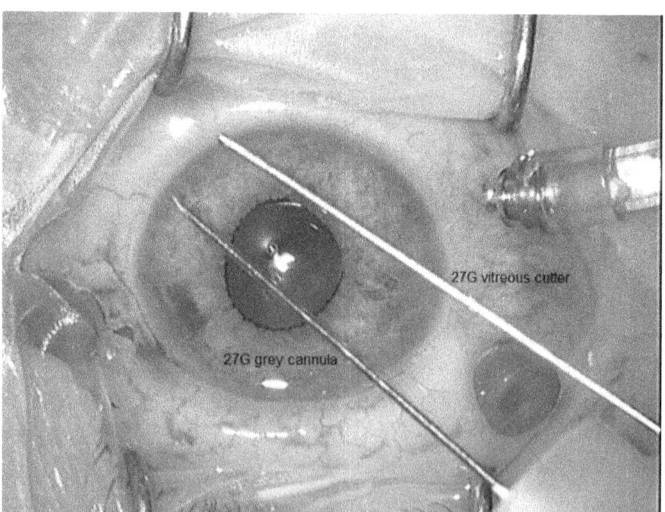

Fig. 7.3 We prefer 27G for easy and difficult cases because the 27G cutter can be used for delamination of membranes. Almost all instruments are nowadays available for 27G except a few

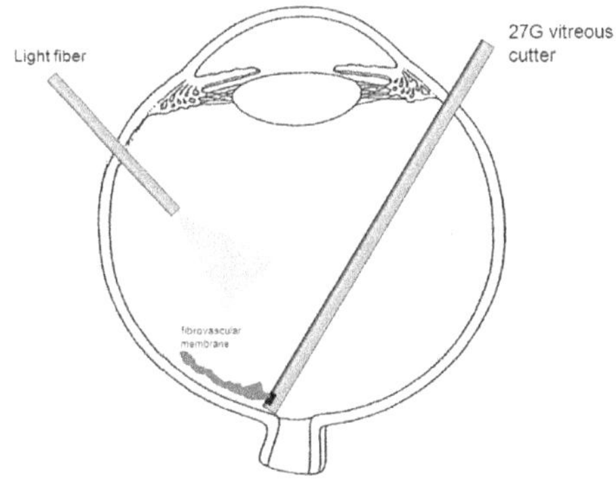

Fig. 7.4 The advantage of the 27G vitreous cutter is that it can be used very close to the retina and can even assist in removing membranes

Surgical pearls
Choice of gauge: Take into account your presurgical assessment and treatment planning for selecting the instruments you will need for this specific diabetic eye. If the eye has extensive fibrovascular membranes, then use a 25G/27G hybrid system. In case of an easy diabetic vitrectomy, we prefer 27G.

7.7.1 Monomanual Vitrectomy

Monomanual vitrectomy is possible in easy cases (Figs. 7.5 and 7.6). Monomanual peeling, however, is difficult in severe or advanced cases because the delamination of the membranes often requires two hands. The 27G vitreous cutter allows a delicate manipulation of the fibrovascular membrane because the instrument can be manoeuvred very close to the retina (Fig. 8.2); if a complete removal is not possible then the membrane can be trimmed down. The trimming is sufficient if the tractive componets of the membranes are removed.

Remark: Monomanual vitrectomy is sufficient for cases with a detached vitreous and hemorrhage. But monomanual vitrectomy has its own limitation in complicated cases with attached posterior vitreous and fibrovascular membranes.

7.7.2 Bimanual Vitrectomy

Bimanual vitrectomy is an essential part of modern Minimal Incision Vitreoretinal Surgery (MIVS). By inserting a stationary chandelier light in the sclera (4-port vitrectomy, Fig. 7.7) the surgeon has two active hands. To operate with two active hands is an essential method for diabetic vitrectomy. We work bimanual throughout all difficult diabetic cases. We perform a bimanual vitrectomy by indenting the sclera with the sclera depressor. The removal of fibrovascular membranes is the

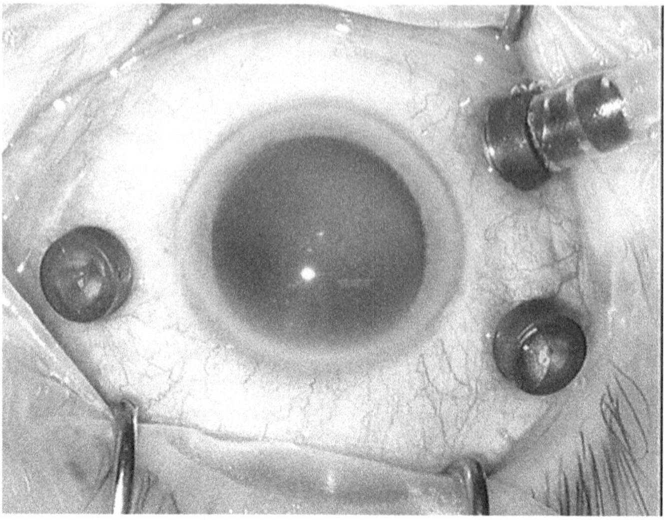

Fig. 7.5 A typical 3-port vitrectomy setup. Be aware that monomanual vitrectomy has clear limitations in diabetic eyes

Fig. 7.6 Monomanual vitrectomy with a handheld light pipe and a vitreous cutter. Be observant that one hand is occupied holding a light pipe. A PRP up to the ora serrata is not possible with monomanual vitrectomy unless the assistant indents the sclera. We discourage indentation by an assistant

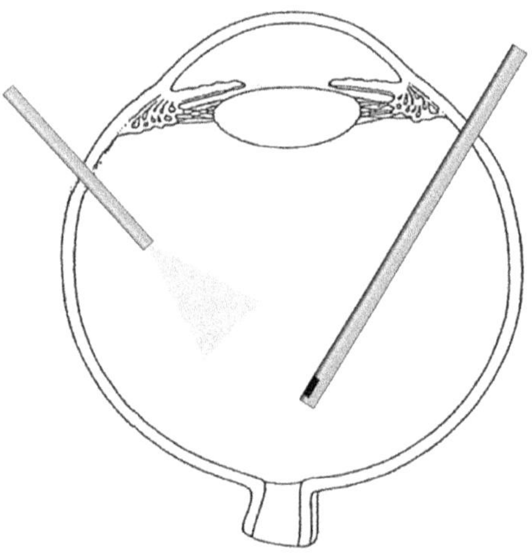

most important surgical part and is much easier when performed bimanual; one hand lifts the membrane and the other delaminates it. Hemostasis is much easier bimanual; one hand aspirates the blood, and the other hand cauterizes the vessel. Even PRP is much easier bimanually enabling a PRP up to the ora serrata with one hand depressing the retinal periphery and the other manoeuvring endolaser probe (Fig. 7.8).

Remark: An alternative to bimanual PRP is an illuminated laser probe. The latter gives, however, only a small light cone whereas a chandelier light illuminates the

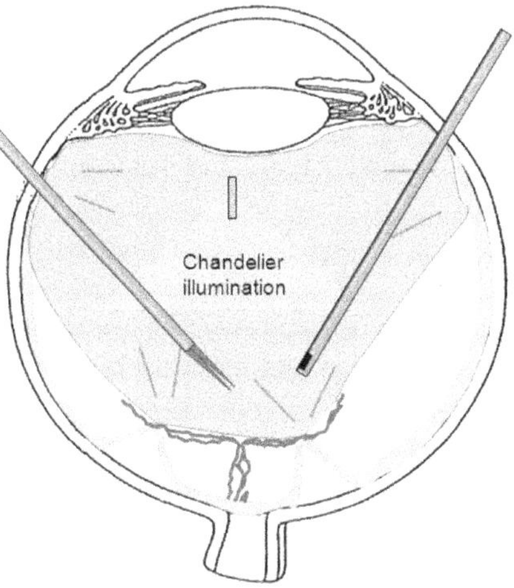

Fig. 7.7 An optimal chandelier illumination gives a 135° panoramic view. Both hands can be used for surgery and especially for the delamination of the fibrovascular membranes

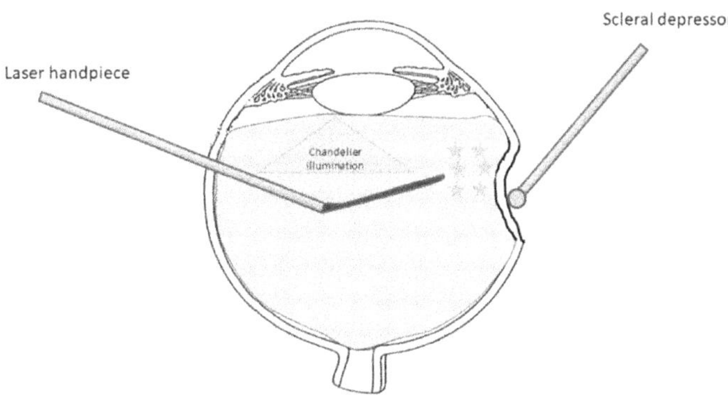

Fig. 7.8 An optimal chandelier illumination enables a fast and complete laser photocoagulation up to the ora serrata. No one indents as well as your two hands

complete retina allowing an easy and fast laser treatment. Remember: No one can indent as good as your second hand.

Surgical pearls

Chandelier light: Try to use chandelier lights in your uncomplicated cases in order to practice their insertion and to trim the vitreous base bimanually with scleral depressor and vitreous cutter. This practice will help when you really need them in challenging cases.

7.8 Take Home Message: Ten Recommendations for VR Surgery of TRD Secondary to Diabetes

(1) Never operate in an angry PDR, make it quiescent before surgery.
(2) Pretreat the eye with anti-VEGF and laser (if possible) and schedule a delayed vitrectomy.
(3) Be generous with laser and anti-VEGF, be hesitant with vitrectomy and avoid cryopexy.
(4) Avoid a combined phaco/vitrectomy in a diabetic eye. Perform first a phaco with Avastin injection and schedule a delayed vitrectomy (two-step approach).
(5) Avoid a monomanual vitrectomy. Prefer a bimanual vitrectomy with chandelier light with special instruments.
(6) The special instruments are intravitreal scissors, a 27G vitreous cutter (alternative: vertical scissors) and a knob spatula (alternative: backflush cannula with silicone tip).
(7) The aim of vitrectomy is the removal of posterior hyaloid with the membranes (PVD).
(8) At the end of vitrectomy always perform a complete panretinal laser photocoagulation (PRP) and inject anti- VEGF.
(9) Prefer a gas tamponade. If you choose a silicone oil tamponade then remove it after maximum of three months.
(10) Don't forget the fellow eye. Treat always both eyes at the same time.

References

Early photocoagulation for diabetic retinopathy. ETDRS report number 9. Early Treatment Diabetic Retinopathy Study Research Group. Ophthalmology. 1991; 98(5 Suppl):766–85. PMID: 2062512.

Obeid A, Su D, Patel SN, Uhr JH, Borkar D, Gao X, Fineman MS, Regillo CD, Maguire JI, Garg SJ, Hsu J. Outcomes of eyes lost to follow-up with proliferative diabetic retinopathy that received panretinal photocoagulation versus intravitreal anti-vascular endothelial growth factor. Ophthalmology. 2019; 126(3):407–413. https://doi.org/10.1016/j.ophtha.2018.07.027. Epub 2018 Aug 2. PMID: 30077614.

Sun JK, Glassman AR, Beaulieu WT, Stockdale CR, Bressler NM, Flaxel C, Gross JG, Shami M, Jampol LM. Diabetic retinopathy clinical research network. Rationale and application of the protocol S anti-vascular endothelial growth factor algorithm for proliferative diabetic retinopathy. Ophthalmology. 2019; 126(1):87–95. https://doi.org/10.1016/j.ophtha.2018.08.001. Epub 2018 Aug 7. PMID: 30096354; PMCID: PMC6916649.

Part IV

Surgery of Easy Diabetic Retinopathy

All videos of this book are found on the Youtube channel from Ulrich Spandau and playing list ”Proliferative diabetic retinopathy” (link: https://youtube.com/playlist?list=PL0dKYclPD7yM9qRjBoF1HMwtxFfbf2T6A).

Chapter 8 Combined Phaco and anti-VEGF for diabetic eyes (short version)

8.1 Vitreous hemorrhage secondary to PDR

8.2 Easy diabetic case (Audio)

8 Surgery of Easy Diabetic Vitrectomy

8.1 Anaesthesia for Easy Diabetic Vitrectomy

In easy cases such as a PDR with vitreous hemorrhage and no TRD, we use peribulbar anaesthesia. The duration of a vitrectomy is approximately 30–45 minutes.

For peribulbar anaesthesia, we use a blunt retrobulbar cannula (25G, Atkinson, BD) which minimizes the risk to perforate the globe.

We use two different kinds of anaesthesia according to the preference of the surgeon:

(1) Peribulbar anaesthesia: 4 ml solution (e.g., 50% Bupivacaine (Marcain®) and 50% Mepivacaine (Carbocain®)) inferotemporal and 3 ml superior at 12 o'clock next to the eyeball. Then we apply ocular compression for 10 minutes.
(2) Combination of peribulbar and subtenon anaesthesia: 4 ml solution (e.g., 50% Bupivacaine (Marcain®) and 50% Mepivacaine (Carbocain®)) inferotemporal. Then we apply ocular compression for 10 minutes. Under sterile conditions, we then open the conjunctiva and tenon inferonasally and inject with a subtenon cannula 3 ml of solution.

8.2 Treatment Planning for Easy Diabetic Vitrectomy

The treatment planning has already been explained in detail. We will only show once more the treatment algorithm for an easy diabetic vitrectomy (Fig. 8.1). The essential point is that you perform a vitrectomy in a pseudophakic eye.

U. Spandau and Z. Tomic, *Small-Gauge Vitrectomy for Diabetic Retinopathy*,
https://doi.org/10.1007/978-3-031-26204-3_8

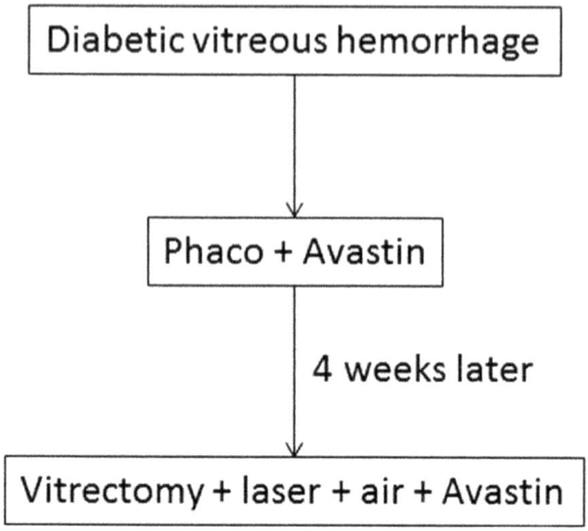

Fig. 8.1 Our treatment algorithm for treatment planning of a PDR for an old type 2 diabetic

8.3 Sequential Phacoemulsification and Anti-VEGF Treatment

A two-step phacoemulsification/vitrectomy is essential to reduce postoperative inflammation and vitreous hemorrhage. Perform a phacoemulsification as usual. Inject the IOL and place it into the capsular bag. Before removing the viscoelastics, perform an intravitreal injection with an anti-VEGF medication. Inject 0.1 of anti-VEGF solution. Then remove the viscoelastics and hydrate the incisions (Figs. 8.2 and 8.3).

The surgical video of this technique can be viewed here: 8.0 Combined Phaco Avastin, video link: https://youtu.be/g4rVmn1m_ps.

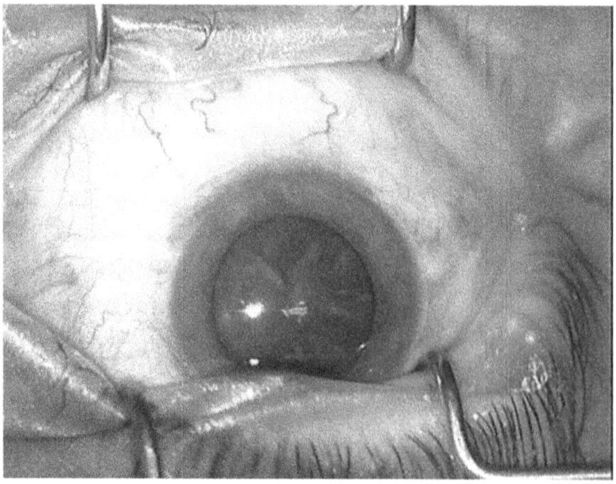

Fig. 8.2 A diabetic eye with vitreous hemorrhage. We apply a stepwise technique: first a combined phacoemulsification with intravitreal Avastin and 1 month later, if still necessary, a vitrectomy

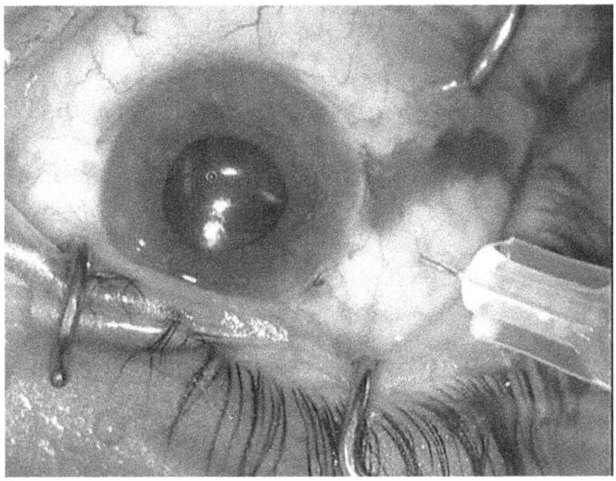

Fig. 8.3 After implantation of the IOL and before removal of the viscoelastics an intravitreal injection of Avastin (0.1 ml) is performed

Surgical pearls
Avoid a lens sparing vitrectomy in a vitreous hemorrhage. Why? Because the anterior vitreous hemorrhage behind the lens cannot be removed as the chance of lens touch is high. But the removal of the anterior vitreous is essential because it reduces the incidence of postoperative hemorrhage and the risk for a PVR detachment.

8.4 Easy Diabetic Vitrectomy

8.4.1 Introduction

A vitreous hemorrhage with attached retina and no associated major vitreoretinal pathology is suitable for the beginner. In most cases, a PVD is present and the hemorrhage fills out the vitreous gel behind the lens. In the presence of vitreous hemorrhage, a previous history of panretinal photocoagulation usually facilitates the surgery, because it is associated with a higher rate of posterior vitreous detachment and promotes retinal adhesion to the RPE and choroid. He/she learns to work with the vitreous cutter and apply a PRP, but does not need to perform any significant manipulations of the retina.

The main problem with this procedure is that there is no view of the fundus (Fig. 8.4). The procedure is even harder when the natural lens is still present, due to the risk of injuring the posterior capsule. Perform, therefore, PPVs only in pseudophakic eyes.

Practice the application of panretinal laser photocoagulation (PRP) very well using a chandelier light. In one hand, hold the scleral depressor and indent the sclera and retina, and in the other hand, hold the laser probe and apply a PRP up to the ora serrata. This surgery can be performed under local anaesthesia. We use mostly 25G and 27G for these cases. The surgical video of this technique can be viewed here: 8.1 Easy diabetic vitrectomy.

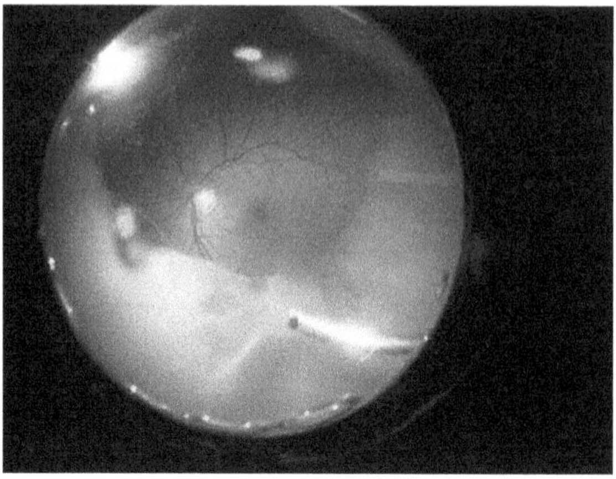

Fig. 8.4 A dense vitreous hemorrhage with detached posterior vitreous

Surgical pearls

B-scan: In cases with vitreous hemorrhage, always perform a detailed preoperative ultrasound examination. Try to determine the state of the posterior vitreous face (attached, partially attached or detached) and the retina.

8.4.2 Surgery

Instruments

1. **25G and 27G 3-port trocar system with or without chandelier illumination**
2. **120D lens**
3. **Vitreous cutter**
4. **Backflush instrument**
5. **Scleral depressor.**

Tamponade

Air, SF_6

Individual steps

1. **3-port trocar system with or without chandelier illumination**
2. **Core vitrectomy**
3. **Peripheral vitrectomy**
4. **PRP up to ora serrata**
5. **Fluid x air exchange and intravitreal anti-VEGF treatment**
6. **Tamponade and removal of the trocar cannulas.**

The surgery step-by-step:

1. 3-port trocar system with chandelier illumination

2. Core vitrectomy

The vitreous hemorrhage reduces the illumination of the light fibre, because the light cone is hidden by blood. Therefore, the surgeon should first make a core vitrectomy. Keep the vitreous cutter behind the IOL and remove all vitreous gel. It might be easier to work first without BIOM and use the microscope only as you would in cataract surgery. If the visibility is not improved, then try only to aspirate the liquefied blood. Try next to cut a break in the posterior hyaloid in order to obtain a view of the fundus (Fig. 8.4). It is important to identify the retinal vessels to make sure that the surgeon is in the right plane (and not in the subretinal space). If successful, continue the vitrectomy from the break into the posterior hyaloid.

Surgical pearls

Blocked infusion: The hemorrhagic vitreous blocks sometimes the infusion. Check the infusion trocar before vitrectomy and if in doubt then cut the hemorrhagic vitreous around the infusion trocar.

3. Peripheral vitrectomy

Proceed to trim the vitreous base. Do not trim the vitreous base completely because the risk of causing damage to the retina is higher than the benefits. If the posterior vitreous body is not detached, then a PVD should be performed now. If the aetiology of the bleeding is for example a bleeding vessel, treat it now with laser, diathermy or cryo.

Surgical pearls

How should epiretinal blood be removed? 1. Aspirate epiretinal blood by sweeping with a silicone tip flute needle over the retina. 2. By pressing several times on the side opening/tubing of the backflush instrument, water is ejected from the tip of the flute needle and blows the epiretinal blood upward. The blood can then be easily aspirated at the same time with the vitreous cutter. 3. Clotted blood can be grasped with an ILM forceps and be removed with the vitreous cutter.

4. Panretinal photocoagulation (PRP) up to ora serrata

We recommend completing a PRP intraoperatively in all cases of vitrectomy for proliferative diabetic retinopathy. This is the best opportunity to complete the PRP, as rebleeding into the vitreous cavity is a common problem following vitrectomy, which will have a negative influence on performing additional PRP after the vitrectomy. Use the scleral depressor and apply a dense PRP up to the ora serrata (Figs. 8.5, 8.6 and 8.7). After endolaser photocoagulation check if a new hemorrhage occurred at the central pole and treat it before you move on to the tamponade.

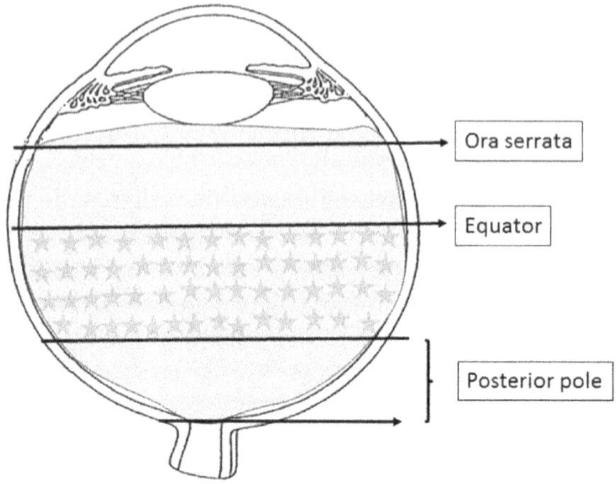

Fig. 8.5 In most cases the retina is only treated up to the equator. There are no laser spots between equator and ora serrata

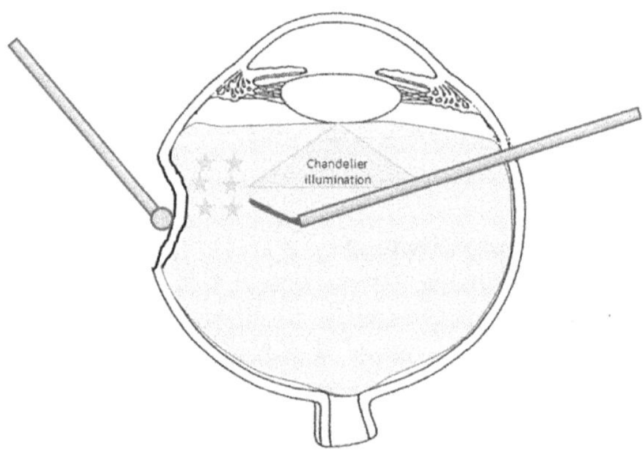

Fig. 8.6 After insertion of a chandelier light a PRP up to the ora serrata can be performed with one hand indenting the sclera and the other hand holding the laser handpiece

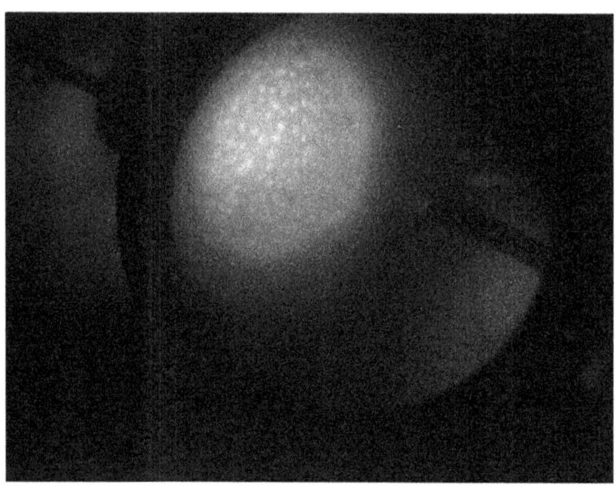

Fig. 8.7 Perform a PRP up to the ora serrata

Surgical pearls

Small pupil: If the pupil constricts during surgery, inject 0.01% Adrenalin into the anterior chamber. The pupil enlarges within seconds. If the small pupil is caused by posterior synechiae, use stretching instruments such as a push–pull or insert iris hooks to enlarge the pupil.

5. Fluid x air exchange and intravitreal anti-VEGF treatment

An air or gas tamponade is recommended to reduce the risk of rebleeding into the vitreous cavity. Perform first a fluid (against) air exchange. Then inject 0.1 to 0.2 ml bevacizumab into the air filled eye.

6. Tamponade and removal of the trocar cannulas

For an easy diabetic vitrectomy, we use in most cases air and sometimes SF_6 as tamponade. Finally the trocars are removed.

8.5 Surgery of Easy Diabetic Vitrectomy Vitrectomy Case with ATTACHED Posterior Hyaloid

The difficulty of surgery of these patients is underestimated because a moderate to severe diabetic retinopathy without tractions is present. The indication may be a vitreous haemorrhage but also can be a VMTS or an epiretinal membrane. After you completed a core vitrectomy you see that the posterior hyaloid is attached (Fig. 8.8). When you start to induce a PVD you realize that the posterior hyaloid is very adherent not only in the posterior pole but up to the ora serrata. This means that you may induce focal detachments with and without ruptures in the periphery. Try to induce cautiously a PVD up to the ora serrata and remove the anterior vitreous completely. We strongly recommend to remove the complete anterior vitreous because the risk for a postoperative anterior PVR is decreased by doing so. This means that the eye should be pseudophakic for the ease of surgery. Perform always a scatter laser upto the ora and add anti-VEGF.

8.6 Complications

Air tamponade: Air does not expand at sea level. But patients with an air tamponade are not allowed to fly because air expands with increasing altitude. The air pressure in the plane corresponds to an air pressure at 2500 m above sea level. Travel to higher elevations should also be avoided.

Recurrent vitreous hemorrhage: After a vitrectomy for a vitreous hemorrhage, bleeding may reoccur after surgery. If the recurrence is associated with a hyphema then check if the patient takes anticoagulants, i.e., aspirin. The patient should stop taking blood thinning medication for approximately 1 month. In most cases, the hyphema resolves. Do not reoperate on the patient before the hyphema has resolved.

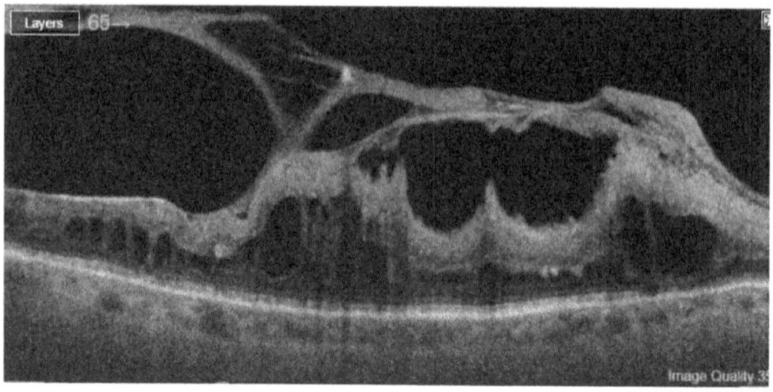

Fig. 8.8 OCT showing strong adhesions between the posterior hyaloid and the retina in an 83 y/o diabetic patient with type 2 diabetes

8.7 FAQ

Do you peel the ILM in diabetic retinopathy?

No, never. The only exception would be a very difficult case complicated by PVR. There are no double-blind studies published which support the prophylactic removal of physiologic tissue such as ILM.

Part V

Surgery of Difficult Diabetic Vitrectomy

All videos of this book are found on the Youtube channel from Ulrich Spandau and playing list "Proliferative diabetic retinopathy" (link: https://youtube.com/playlist?list=PL0dKYclPD7yM9qRjBoF1HMwtxFfbf2T6A).

Chapter 10:

10.1 Diabetic retinopathy_audio

10.2 PVD_induction

10.3 PVD no blood

10.4 PVD with_blood

10.5 Bimanual peeling with brush and forceps

10.6 Bimanual_peeling_with_knob spatula

10.7 Bimanual_peeling_with_scissors

10.8 Bimanual peeling with scissors_2

10.9 Bimanual_peeling_with_cutter

10.10 Hemostasis for PDR

10.11 Management of strong bleeding with knob spatula

10.12 Laser under PFCL

10.13 Tamponade_Air

10.14 Tamponade_Silicone

Chapter 10: A total retinal detachment secondary to diabetes

Chapter 10: Advanced TRD for diabetic retinopathy

Chapter 10: Advanced proliferative diabetic retinopathy with detachment of posterior pole

Instruments and Surgical Techniques for Difficult Diabetic Vitrectomy

9

9.1 Instruments

A difficult diabetic vitrectomy can only be successfully operated with the right instruments. The essential instruments are (1) backflush instrument with silicone tip, (2) endgripping forceps and (3) intravitreal scissors (curved or straight). Vertical scissors are not sufficient. The individual surgical instruments are introduced here.

9.1.1 Vitreous Cutter

The 27G vitreous cutter from Alcon/DORC is a "game changer" in diabetic vitrectomy. The smaller the vitreous cutter the more it can help you to remove diabetic membranes. Especially 27-gauge vitreous cutters facilitate the dissection and removal of fibrovascular membranes. A good alternative is the bevelled 25G vitreous cutter from Alcon.

9.1.2 Illumination for Bimanual Vitrectomy

Chandelier light fibre
A chandelier light provides a panoramic light source and illuminates the entire fundus. A chandelier light is either fixated directly in the sclera or in a trocar. This enables bimanual surgery and allows the surgeon to use a second active instrument in addition to the vitreous cutter. For optimal illumination of a chandelier light, an external light source (Photon, Xenon) or a modern vitrectomy machine (Stellaris PC, Constellation, Eva) is required.

U. Spandau and Z. Tomic, *Small-Gauge Vitrectomy for Diabetic Retinopathy*,
https://doi.org/10.1007/978-3-031-26204-3_9

9.1.3 Instruments for Hemostasis

Treat retinal bleeding sites with laser. If this is not sufficient, use endodiathermy. If endodiathermy does not help, then compress the source of bleeding 1 minute with a vitreous cutter.

Endodiathermy probe
An endodiathermy is useful for (1) marking of retinal breaks and (2) cauterizing bleeding retinal vessels such as in diabetic retinopathy. There are usually two different types of endodiathermy probes: "Active" endodiathermy probes are combined with a flute needle. This is very useful when treating an acute intraocular hemorrhage. The flute needle drains the hemorrhage, enabling localization of the bleeding site, which can then simultaneously be treated with endodiathermy. "Non-active" diathermy is a straightforward endodiathermy probe with a pointed tip. When treating an acute intraocular hemorrhage you have to work bimanual. One hand holds the endodiathermy probe and the other hand holds the backflush instrument.

9.1.4 Instruments for Peeling of Fibrovascular Membranes

Instruments to fixate the membranes
Backflush instrument (=Charles flute needle), Indication: Fixation of membranes through aspiration of tissue.

Eckardt endgripping forceps
The 27G endgripping forceps from DORC is a mix of ILM forceps and endgripping forceps. It functions well for membranes. We use the 27G forceps for 27G and 25G surgery (DORC, 27G disposable microforceps.1286.WD04).

A good alternative is the 25G and 27G Ultra Peel forceps from DORC (2286.CD304).

Instruments to delaminate the membranes
Knob spatula (Fig. 9.1*)*

The knob spatula has a thick knob at its tip. Indication for use is the manipulation of membranes or a retinal massage. A retinal massage is necessary if there are retinal folds.

Silicone tip flute needle (Fig. 9.2*)*

The flute needle with silicone tip can be used for atraumatic aspiration of fluids close to the retina such as preretinal blood and for delamination of the fibrovascular membrane from the underlying retina; it is an alternative to the knob spatula.

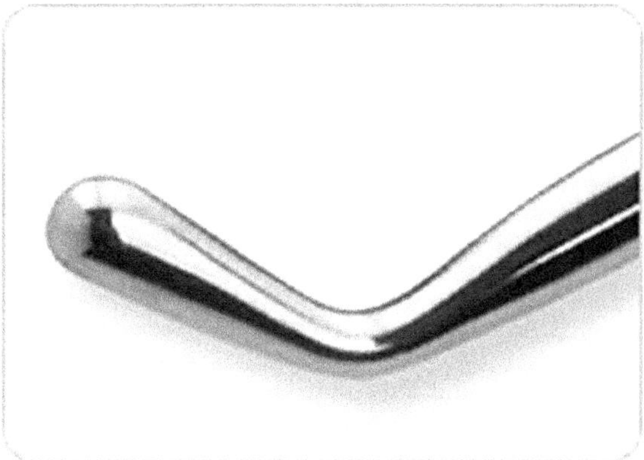

Fig. 9.1 Knob spatula. Available in 23G and 25G. (EyeTechnology, UK: VR-2095)

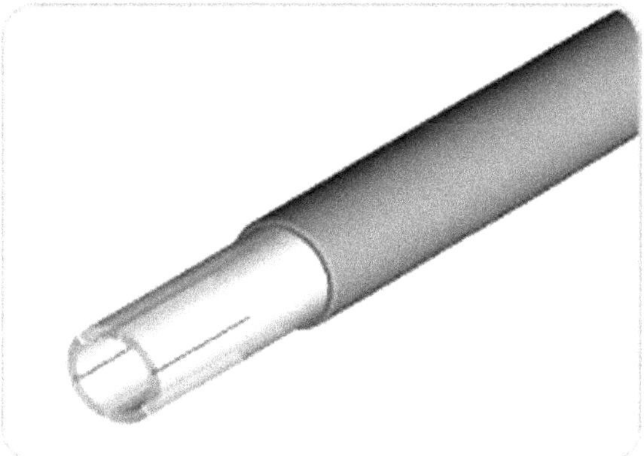

Fig. 9.2 Charles flute needle with silicone tip. We prefer 25G (DORC 2281_AD04)

Membrane pic

The membrane pic is angled at the end. It is very useful for the lifting of membrane edges. A lifted membrane (edge) can then be removed with Eckardt forceps. We recommend the 27G membrane pic from DORC because the small gauge allows an atraumatic delamination of membranes (DORC, 1292.E04).

Instruments to dissect membranes and tissue bridges

Straight horizontal scissors

The horizontal scissors have two straight blades. They are used for dissecting membranes from the retina, i.e., cutting the tissue bridges between the membrane and the retina (Fig. 9.3). They are available in 23G (DORC, Geuder) and 25G (Eye Tech, UK).

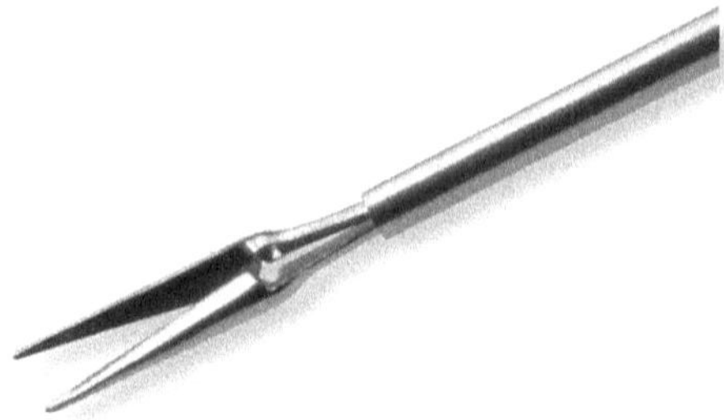

Fig. 9.3 Straight microscissors (25G, Eye Tech, UK)

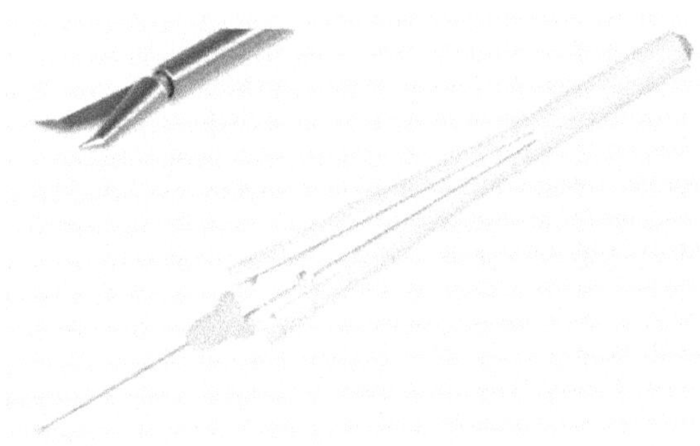

Fig. 9.4 Disposable microscissors, hooked, 27G. DORC: 2286.PD04. A good alternative is reusable straight scissors, 25G, from Eye Tech, UK: VR-1811

*Curved microscissors (*Fig. 9.4*)*

A good alternative is the disposable microscissors from DORC. Available in 23G (DORC 1286.M06), 25G (DORC 1286.MD05) and 27G (2286.PD04). We prefer 27G microscissors.

*Vertical scissors (*Fig. 9.5*)*

These 25-gauge retinectomy scissors have two angled blades. They can be helpful in cutting a membrane in two parts but you cannot cut tissue bridges between the membrane and the retina. An alternative to vertical scissors is the 27G cutter.

9.1.5 Dyes

Dyes are sometimes useful to stain tractional membranes or the vitreous during surgery. If you cannot visualize the tissue (membranes or vitreous) then do not hesitate to stain it with triamcinolone or trypan blue. The dyes are preloaded in syringes which are difficult to manipulate. We inject the dye into regular 3 ml syringes which are easy to use.

Trypan Blue
MonoBlue® (DORC): Indication: Staining of the vitreous and membranes.

Fig. 9.5 Vertical scissors are available in 23G (1286.E06) and 25G (1286.ED05) (DORC)

9.1.6 Instruments for Laser Treatment

Laser probe
Straight or curved laser probes are available. The curved laser is particularly suitable for the peripheral retina; the straight laser is handier for the central posterior pole. If you apply a peripheral laser treatment (break, peripheral ischemic retina), the use of a scleral depressor is recommended, which makes the break more accessible and avoids touching the lens. This can be performed either using a chandelier light and a scleral depressor or using the light pipe as a scleral depressor with transscleral illumination. Alternatively, you can use an illuminated laser fibre.

Scleral depressor
A scleral depressor indents the retina. It is a standard instrument for pars plana vitrectomy. It is used for trimming of the vitreous base, particularly in retinal detachment surgery. With a three-port vitrectomy and chandelier endoillumination, you can use the scleral depressor for bimanual trimming of the vitreous base using the vitreous cutter or for panretinal photocoagulation up to the ora serrata. Remember: No one can indent as good as your second hand.

9.1.7 Summary

The essential instruments for a difficult diabetic vitrectomy are a chandelier light, an intravitreal forceps, an intravitreal scissors and a silicone tip backflush instrument.

9.2 Surgical Techniques for a Difficult Diabetic Vitrectomy

9.2.1 Chandelier Light

The chandelier light is best positioned inferonasally, because here its location does not affect the rotation of the eye (Fig. 9.6). The 12 o'clock or 6 o'clock insertion sites disturb the rotation of the globe and the light fibre is easily dislocated when the globe is rotated upwards or downwards. Some chandelier lights (Synergetics, Alcon) have a rigid cable which allows bending of the light fibre and henceforth the ability to manoeuvre the light to different directions in the vitreous cavity. Only external light sources (photon or xenon) have enough power for a sufficient illumination of the vitreous cavity (Fig. 9.7).

If you have never used a chandelier light before, then start with one which can be inserted in a trocar. The 25-gauge chandelier light from DORC (Fig. 9.8)

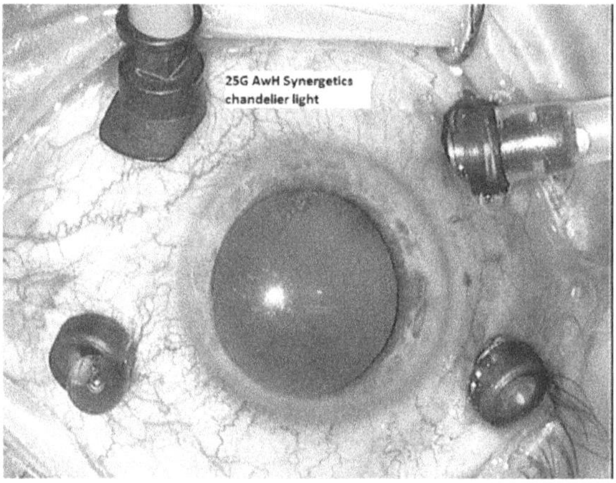

Fig. 9.6 A three-port vitrectomy with chandelier light. This is the typical setup for bimanual vitrectomy. Bimanual vitrectomy is the method of choice for diabetic retinopathy. A 25G Awh chandelier light is used. We prefer the inferonasal position for the chandelier light because this quadrant is not occupied by a trocar. In addition, the eye can be freely rotated without disturbing the chandelier light

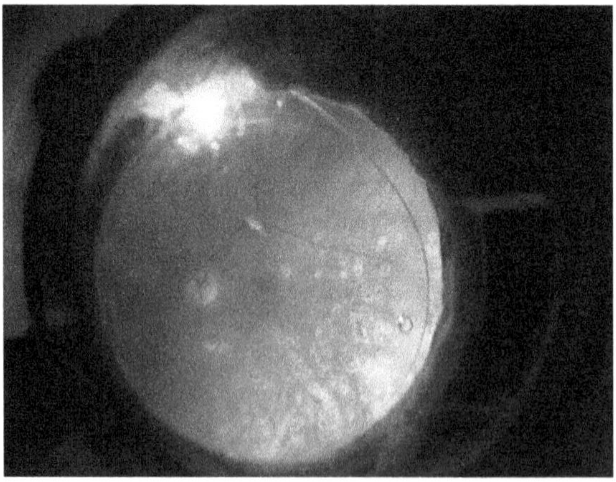

Fig. 9.7 An intraoperative image of a retina illuminated from a Synergetics chandelier light. Find a chandelier light that suits you and use a powerful light source

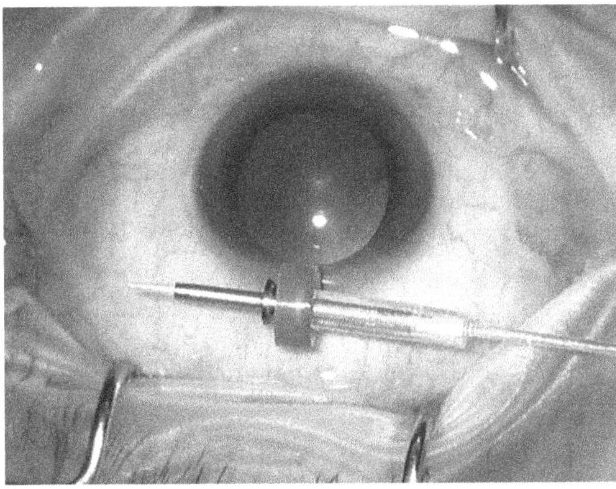

Fig. 9.8 An alternative is a chandelier light from (DORC) which is inserted into the trocar. The light cone is visible on the left side. There is a huge choice of chandelier lights available on the market

is simple to use as the light fibre can be placed inside a regular trocar cannula. Similarly, an Alcon chandelier can also be placed inside a regular trocar cannula.

9.2.2 Posterior Hyaloid Rhexis

The removal of posterior vitreous along with the membranes is the aim of diabetic vitrectomy. It is also the most difficult step of surgery. In a complicated case of proliferative diabetic retinopathy, the posterior hyaloid is always attached at the posterior pole and partially detached in the periphery. In these advanced diabetic retinopathy cases, tractional membranes are present on the posterior pole. If you induce a central PVD, you may be lucky in some cases and the epiretinal neovascularizations will just peel off the retina together with the vitreous face. However, there is a considerable risk of causing major retinal damage by pulling on the membranes and inducing tears in the ischemic and thin retina. Therefore, every case of proliferative diabetic retinopathy should be approached with caution and a PVD should not be induced with the usual method of suction over the posterior pole and pulling on the vitreous face.

Instead, you perform a peripheral PVD (peripheral hyaloidal rhexis). In most cases of proliferative diabetic retinopathy, a partial vitreous detachment is present. This means that the posterior vitreous is still attached centrally but partially detached in the mid-periphery.

Try to find where the peripheral vitreous is detached. Here you create an opening of the posterior hyaloid and remove the vitreous along the posterior vitreous membrane (Figs. 9.9, 9.10, 9.11, 9.12, 9.13 and 9.14) on a constant level in a circular fashion (posterior hyaloid rhexis). In the most cases, a 360° rhexis is not possible because the posterior hyaloid is partially attached (often at the nasal pole) (Figs. 9.9, 9.10, 9.11, 9.12, 9.13 and 9.14). Then remove the posterior hyaloid with the vitreous cutter to the arcades (Figs. 9.13 and 9.14). This technique is called "from periphery to the disc" technique *or* "outside-in technique" (Fig. 10B).

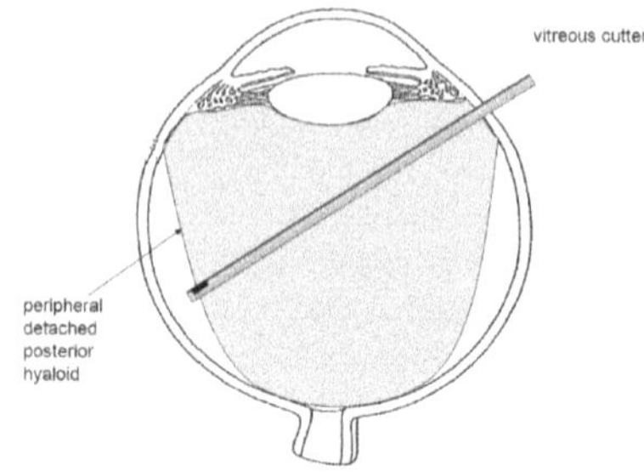

Fig. 9.9 Posterior vitreous rhexis. The posterior hyaloid must be detached in the periphery (not necessarily 360°). This technique cannot be applied if the posterior hyaloid is attached in the periphery, i.e., if no PVD is present

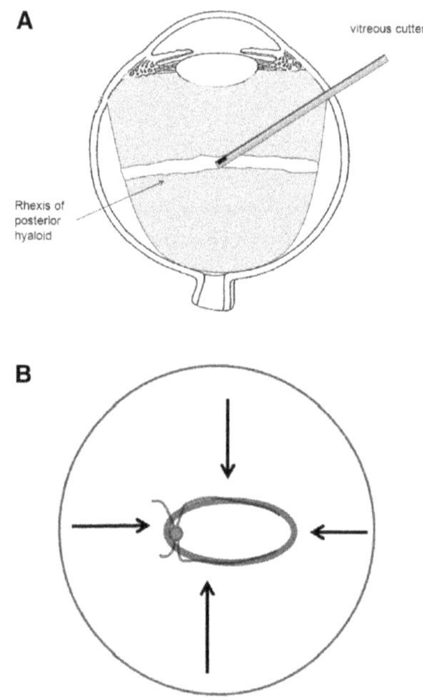

Fig. 9.10 **A** Perform an opening of the posterior hyaloid on the height of the equator. The posterior hyaloid is usually not 360° detached in the periphery. Perform therefore a posterior vitreous rhexis only in that part in which it is detached **B** The recommended technique for membrane removal in diabetic eyes is called "from periphery to the disc" technique *or* "outside-in technique". You start in the periphery and work your way to the optic disc

Remark: This technique is in contrast to membrane peeling in PVR detachment; in the latter an inside-out technique is preferred. Though many surgeons prefer inside-out delamination because the view is better centrally and the central retina is thick and redundant (redundancy because of TRD), we prefer outside-in delamination due to the ease of surgery in getting an edge to start and in manipulating the instruments.

9.2.3 Posterior Vitreous Separation

It may happen that the posterior hyaloid is completely attached and stretches over the posterior pole. An access from the edge of the posterior hyaloid may not be possible. In this case, the opening of this posterior hyaloid is tricky because neither

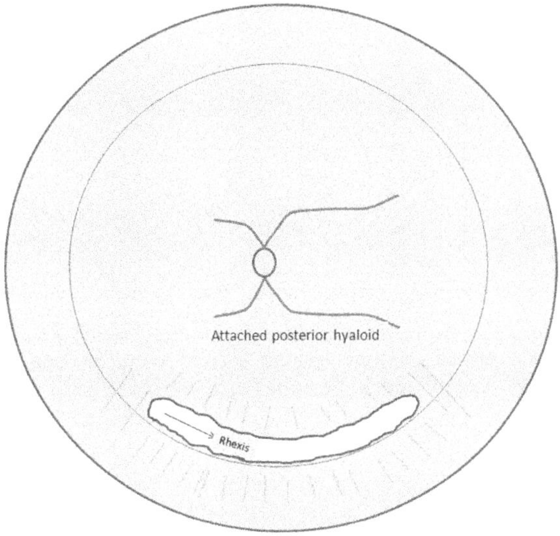

Fig. 9.11 The same procedure seen from a different angle. The posterior hyaloid is attached at the posterior pole and (partially) in the periphery. Begin with a posterior vitreous rhexis on the height of the equator where it is mostly detached

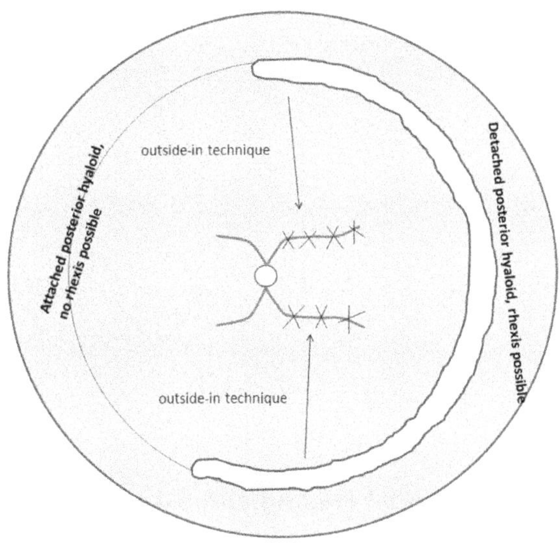

Fig. 9.12 Then continue with the posterior vitreous rhexis circumferentially (in the periphery) where PVD is present. Work from outside to inside (peripheral to central)

the vitreous cutter nor a forceps can grasp the attached posterior hyaloid. The trick is to pierce a hole through the posterior hyaloid. We use the retinal scraper Atkinson retrobulbar blunt needle (Fig. 9.15) for this procedure. Try to open the posterior hyaloid with careful scraping (Figs. 9.16 and 9.17). If you do not succeed then use a regular 27G sharp cannula needle, but the handling of this sharp needle requires more caution.

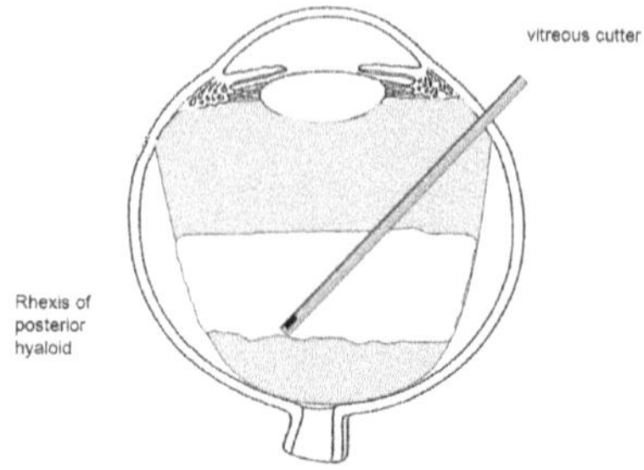

Fig. 9.13 Then remove the vitreous posteriorly up to the temporal arcades, i.e., until you are close to the fibrovascular membranes. Reduce the aspiration of the cutter when you are close to the membranes. Do not pull at the membranes when cutting the vitreous cortex, you may create retinal tears

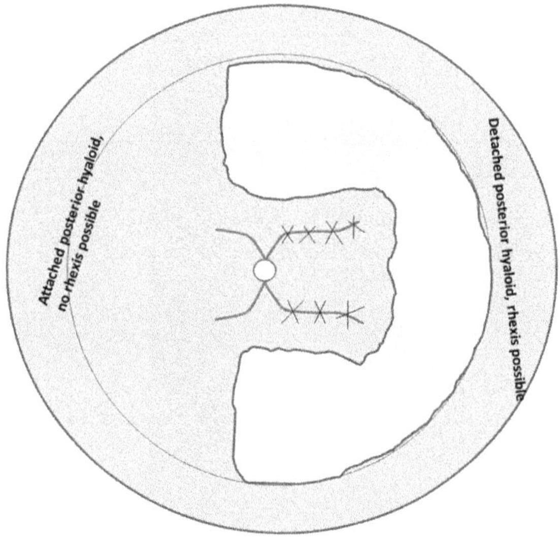

Fig. 9.14 Continue with the removal of the vitreous cortex and hyaloid up to the temporal and nasal arcades. The posterior vitreous of the nasal pole is often attached

9.2.4 Bimanual Peeling and Essential Instruments

The removal of the central posterior hyaloid together with the fibrovascular membranes is technically very challenging. A bimanual peeling of the membranes is technically much easier than a monomanual peeling. Only the use of a chandelier light enables a bimanual peeling. And bimanual peeling enables the surgeon to completely remove the fibrovascular membranes. Switch to bimanual surgery in order to remove the central hyaloid together with the membranes.

Important remark: The most essential instruments for bimanual peeling for tractional detachments are

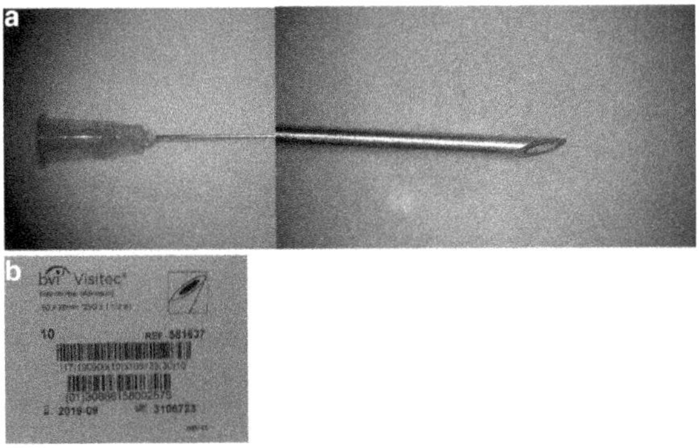

Fig. 9.15 **A, B:** Retinal scraper (25G or 27G retrobulbar cannula Atkinson).This blunt cannula is suitable for opening of the posterior hyaloid or delamination of flat membranes (**A**, **B**). The membrane can be lifted up with this blunt cannula and then be removed with the microforceps. Beaver Visitec, 27G retrobulbar cannula Atkinson

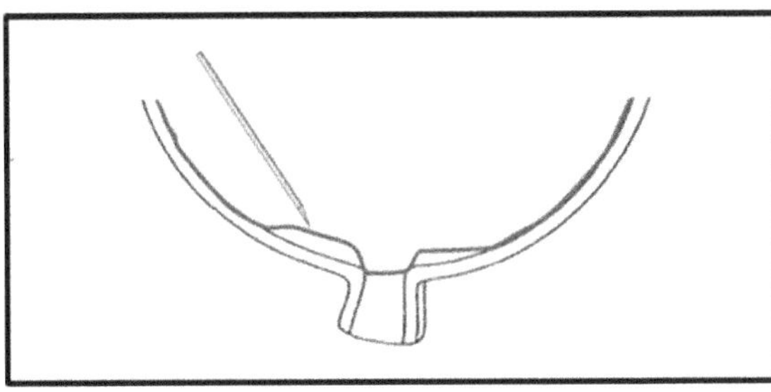

Fig. 9.16 The posterior hyaloid is attached in the periphery and a little bit detached centrally. Pierce a hole in the posterior hyaloid with a 27G needle cannula or a 27G blunt cannula (Atkinson, B&D)

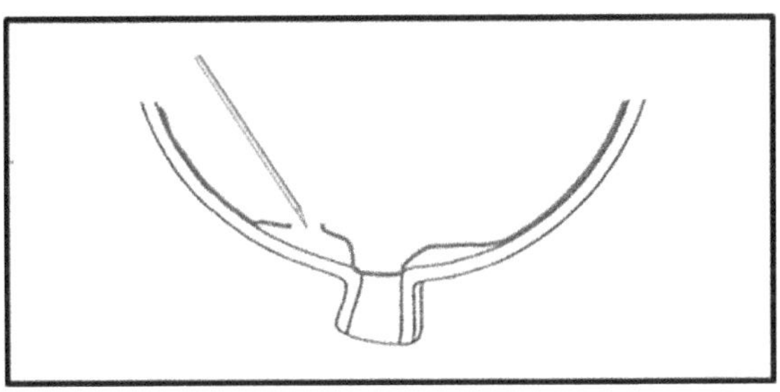

Fig. 9.17 Then you can create a PVD with a forceps or a vitreous cutter. The Atkinson cannula (25G and 27G) is also suitable for delamination of membranes

1. Chandelier light.
2. Intravitreal scissors.
3. Backflush instrument with silicone tip.
4. Endgripping forceps.

If you lack one of these instruments, then do not start surgery.

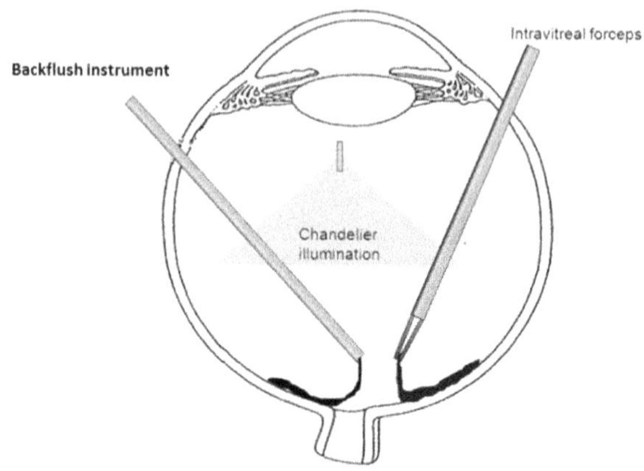

Fig. 9.18 Fixation of membranes. The membrane can be lifted up with a backflush instrument (without silicone tip) in passive aspiration function. The membrane can also be lifted up with a conventional endgripping forceps. The advantage of the backflush instrument is that it releases the membrane when too much force is exerted

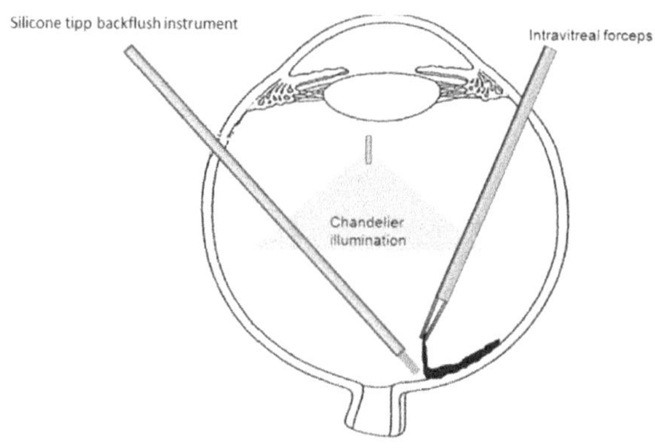

Fig. 9.19 Delamination of membranes. The membrane is delaminated from the retina with a backflush instrument with silicone tip

Use a backflush instrument without silicone tip or an endgripping forceps to lift up the membranes from the underlying retina (Fig. 9.18). This procedure requires *blunt* delamination. Use a backflush instrument with silicone tip or a knob spatula to delaminate the membranes from the underlying retina (Fig. 9.19). Use intravitreal curved or straight scissors to cut the adhesions between the membranes and the underlying retina (Fig. 9.20). Tissue bridges between the membrane attachment pegs can be cut into two parts with vertical scissors or a vitreous cutter (Fig. 9.21). Membrane removal implies a constant switch between delamination and segmentation (Fig. 9.22) and subsequently removal in pieces. Segmentation now is mostly used to find a different access site for the delamination.

9.2.5 Removal of Membranes Located on the Vessel Arcade

The removal of large adherent membranes located on the big vessels is dangerous and can lead to damage of the blood vessels. Start to dissect the membrane outside of the vessels and try then to remove the membrane from the underlying big

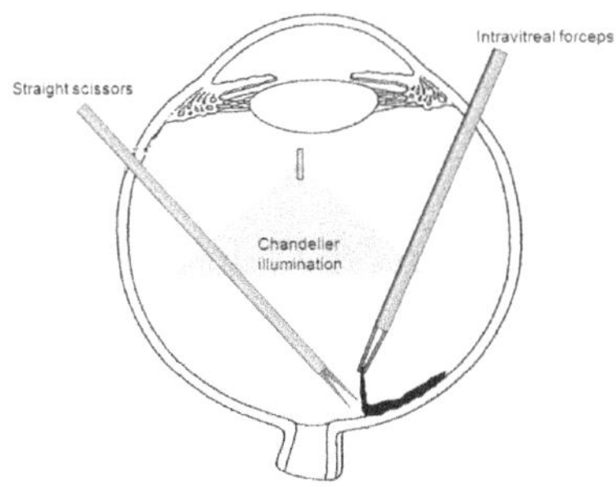

Fig. 9.20 **Dissection of membranes.** The adhesions between the membrane and retina are cut with intravitreal scissors. The membrane should be pulled parallel to the retina

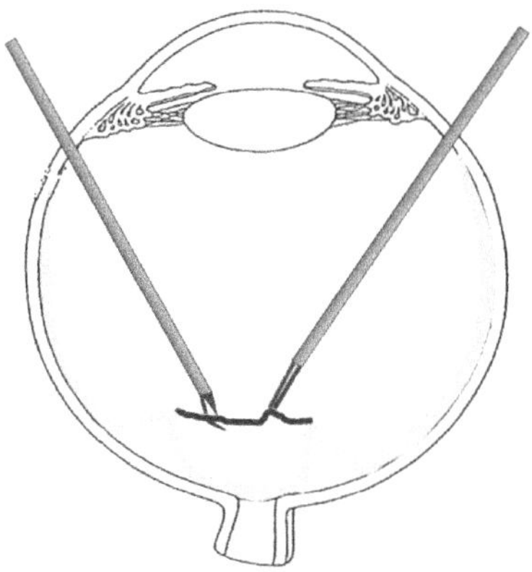

Fig. 9.21 **Cutting of tissue bridge.** A tissue bridge is lifted up gently with an endgripping forceps and cut with vertical scissors. Alternatively, you can use a 27G vitreous cutter (Alcon, DORC) or a 25G bevel vitreous cutter (Alcon)

vessels. If there is too much adherence, trim the membrane from the surrounding tissue and release the anteroposterior tractional components thereby decreasing the pull on the retina and big vessels.

9.2.6 Hemostasis

The best method to prevent intraoperative bleeding is a pretreatment of the eye with anti-VEGF and laser before surgery. Raised arterial blood pressure, valsalva manoeuvre, coughing, hypothermia during anaesthesia and positive pressure ventilation all contribute to increased chances of intraocular bleeding. Diabetic end stage renal disease with uraemia may have deranged coagulation mechanism. Renal dialysis with heparin further increases the chance of bleeding.

There are several methods to reduce retinal hemorrhages:

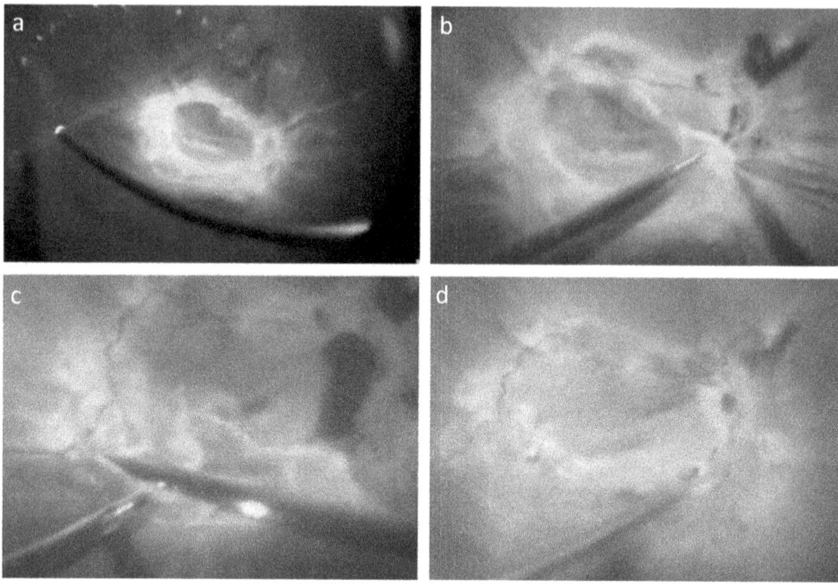

Fig. 9.22 **a–d** A surgical sequence of removal of the fibrovascular membranes. Note the minimal amount of bleeding after 4 weeks of Avastin treatment

(1) **Bottle up:** Increase the intraocular pressure to approximately 40–60 mmHg. Be cautious about the diastolic blood pressure if DBP is lower than the elevated pressure (e.g., in hypotensive general anaesthesia), it can cause ischemic optic neuropathy in an already compromised optic nerve. High IOP can be kept for a maximum of 3 minutes in compromised retina but the best practise is not to exceed 1 minute at a time. Though most retinal surgeons hesitate to elevate IOP above arterial pressure (spontaneous arterial pulsation seen), Hilton GF observed that retina may be able to tolerate occlusion of central retinal artery for 10 minutes (Hilton 1986).
(2) **Laser:** Aspirate the blood with the flute needle and treat the bleeding source with laser in the fellow hand (Fig. 9.23); this technique is especially recommended for bleedings within the temporal arcade.
(3) **Endodiathermy:** Endodiathermy is done bimanually. Aspirate the blood with the flute needle and cauterize the bleeding source with minimal endodiathermy (Fig. 9.24). Heavy diathermy can cause sub-clinical thermal necrosis of retinal tissue leading to a late atrophic break or even bleeding. This technique is recommended for bleedings outside the temporal arcade.
(4) **Vitreous cutter:** Compress the bleeding source for 1 minute with the vitreous cutter or the knob spatula (Fig. 9.25).
(5) **Adrenaline:** Add adrenaline to the BSS plus bottle, especially for diffuse bleeding (0.1–0.3 ml of 1:1000 in 500 ml of BSS Plus). You may get a rebound bleed postoperative once the effect of adrenaline is gone. In very ischemic

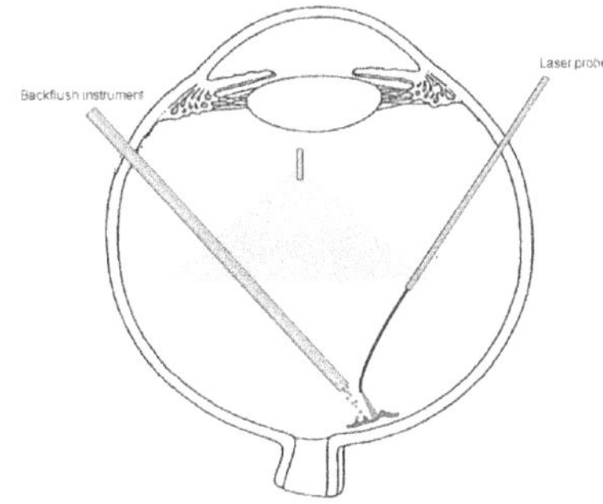

Fig. 9.23 Bimanual hemostasis with a laser probe. One hand holds the backflush instrument and aspirates the blood, and the fellow hand coagulates the bleeding source

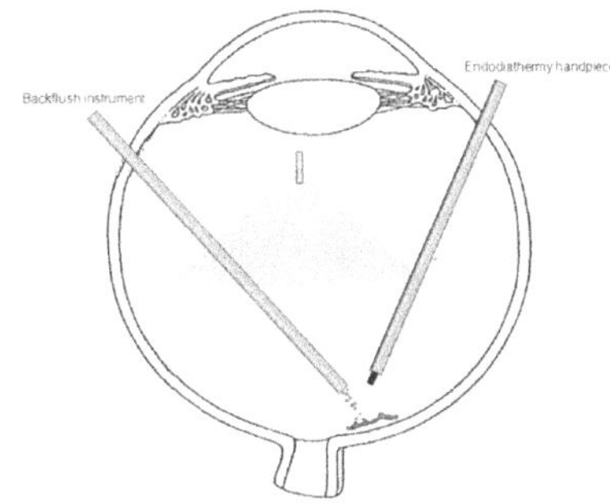

Fig. 9.24 Bimanual hemostasis with Charles flute needle and endodiathermy

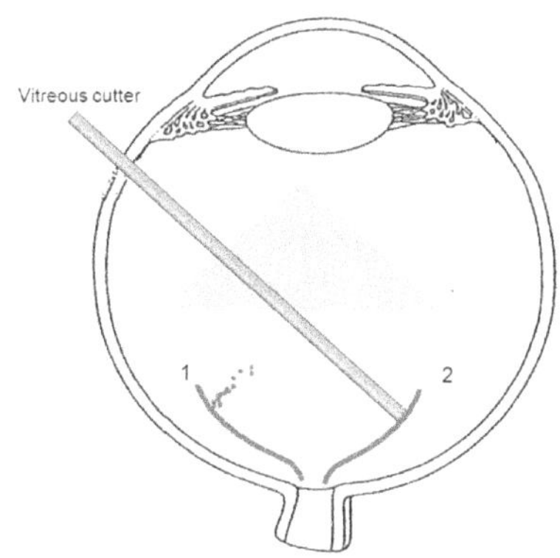

Fig. 9.25 Mechanical hemostasis. Compress the bleeding source for 1 minute with a knob spatula or a vitreous cutter. 1 = bleeding retinal vessel. 2 = compression of bleeding vessel

retina, avoid adrenaline as it promotes vasoconstriction and vasocompromise. Caution advised in ischemic heart disease and high systolic blood pressure. Avoid BSS as it contains citrate which has anticoagulant property. Instead use BSS Plus.

(6) **Fluid-air exchange:** If the bleeding is so severe that there is no view, then you should perform a fluid-air exchange. Then try to visualize and cauterize the bleeding source.

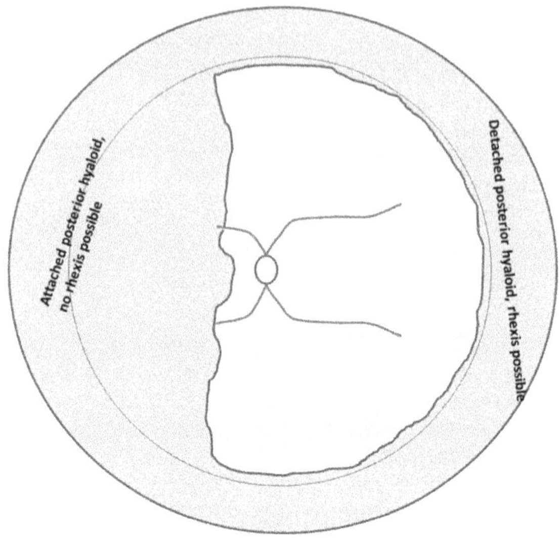

Fig. 9.26 In a final step the remaining attached posterior hyaloid is removed. This is often the case in the nasal quadrant. This may be easy, but in many cases a bimanual delamination is required due to retinal adhesions

9.2.7 Injection of PFCL

In case of a retinal detachment PFCL is required to flatten the retina. Inject PFCL up to the equator. The presence of posterior PFCL also facilitates the subsequent removal of anterior membranes. After removal of all membranes, PFCL is injected up to the ora serrata in order to facilitate a scatter laser treatment.

9.2.8 Posterior Hyaloid Removal on the Nasal Pole

The posterior hyaloid is often attached at the posterior pole. Remove finally the residual attached posterior hyaloid (if present) up to the vitreous base (Figs. 9.26 and 9.27). A bimanual approach is required.

9.2.9 Scatter Laser Treatment

A scatter laser treatment is the most important step for diabetic vitrectomy. Laser photocoagulation destroys retinal tissue, downregulates the expression of VEGF and stops the proliferation of retinal vessels. Furthermore, laser increases diffusion of oxygen from choroid to retina through the atrophic chorioretinal scars. By destroying the peripheral retina, it also decreases the oxygen requirement of the periphery and thereby allows a better oxygenation of the posterior pole. A laser photocoagulation from the arcades to the ora serrata is required. A laser photocoagulation from the arcades to the equator is not sufficient. Why? Thorough ablation of the peripheral retina up to the ora serrata leaves little chance of VEGF production by these ischemic tissues and hence achieves stabilization early. Eyes which

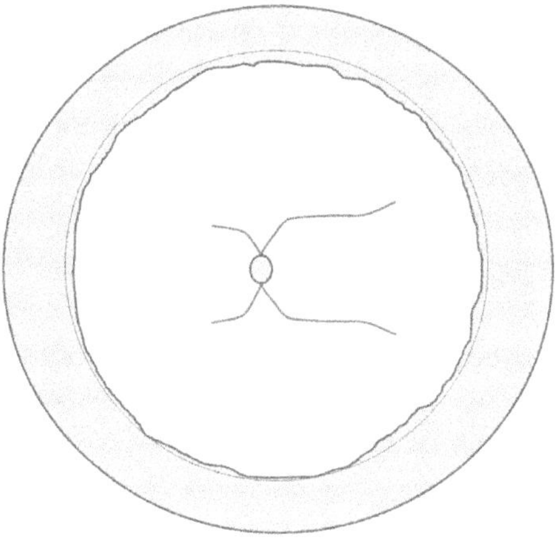

Fig. 9.27 This is the final status. The complete posterior hyaloid and all membranes are removed

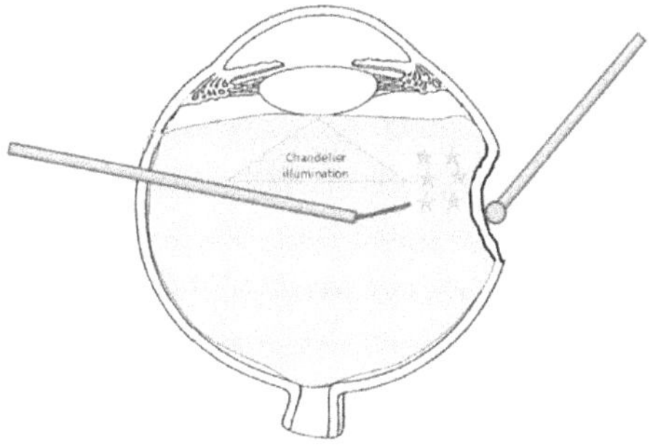

Fig. 9.28 Bimanual laser photocoagulation. One hand indents the sclera and the other hand laser treats the retina up to the ora serrata

receive a scatter laser from the medical retina department are only treated up to the equator and sometimes retinal blood vessels form at the border of treated and non-treated retina. The only way to stop the proliferations in these eyes is the laser treatment up to the ora serrata. Laser coagulation is always performed bimanual in order to reach the ora serrata (Fig. 9.28). If the retina is detached then PFCL is required to flatten the retina. If the retina is attached then laser photocoagulation is performed under BSS.

9.2.9.1 Choice of Tamponade: Gas or Silicone Oil

As tamponade we use mostly a gas tamponade and rarely a silicone oil tamponade. The advantage of the gas is that it absorbs on its own and that it has a higher surface tension which reduces postoperative hemorrhage. The advantage of silicone oil is a clear view to fundus. The disadvantage of silicone oil is emulsification, secondary glaucoma and the necessity of a second surgery. In addition, silicone oil is disadvantageous if there is a postoperative cavity hemorrhage. The bleeding gets compartmentalized under oil as compared to being diffuse in BSS or gas-filled eyes and compartmentalized hemorrhage absorbs very slowly and sometimes becomes difficult to remove off the retina after initial surgery without tearing the retina. So, if you choose silicone oil as tamponade then remove it after 3 months. If you have no breaks and no residual traction, we use an air tamponade. If breaks are present but no residual traction, we use 20% Sf6. In difficult cases (more bleeding, only eye, breaks and residual tractions are present) we use silicone oil.

Reference

Hilton GF. Planned elevation of intraocular pressure with temporary occlusion of the central retinal artery during retinal surgery. Arch Ophthalmol. 1986;104(7):975. https://doi.org/10.1001/archopht.1986.01050190033019. PMID: 3729790.

Surgery of Difficult Diabetic Vitrectomy

10

10.1 Anaesthesia for Difficult Diabetic Vitrectomy

Difficult cases are usually operated on under general anaesthesia, particularly in young patients with insulin-dependent diabetes. The duration of a vitrectomy in difficult cases is approximately 90–120 minutes.

10.2 Treatment Planning for Difficult Diabetic Vitrectomy

The main features of a difficult diabetic vitrectomy case are a partial scatter laser-treated retina, a tractional retinal detachment and a partial PVD in the periphery. The treatment planning is shown in Diagram 10.1. First, we start with an anti-VEGF injection. Then we schedule a laser treatment or a vitrectomy. We always treat the fellow eye at the same time either with laser or with anti-VEGF. *Remark:* Pretreated means the eye was treated with partial/incomplete scatter laser prior to vitrectomy.

The surgical technique for a difficult diabetic vitrectomy case is an "outside-inside" technique. This means that we remove the posterior vitreous from the periphery to the central pole.

10.3 Difficult Diabetic Vitrectomy

Instruments

1. **25G/27G three-port trocar system with chandelier illumination.**
2. **120D lens, for central peeling: 60D lens.**
3. **Vitreous cutter.**
4. **Backflush instrument.**

U. Spandau and Z. Tomic, *Small-Gauge Vitrectomy for Diabetic Retinopathy*,
https://doi.org/10.1007/978-3-031-26204-3_10

Diagram 10.1 Our surgical algorithm for a pretreated diabetic vitrectomy case

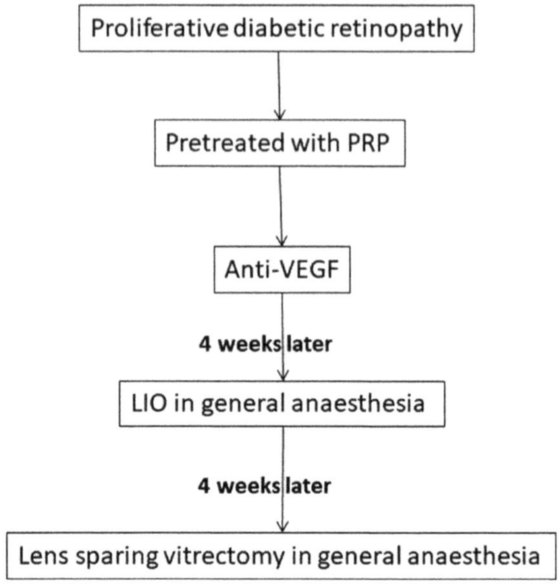

5. 27G endgripping forceps (DORC).
6. 27G curved scissors (DORC).
7. Silicone tip Charles flute needle with silicone tip (vacuum cleaner).
8. Endodiathermy (DORC, Alcon).
9. Laser probe.
10. Scleral depressor.

Maybe:

25G straight scissors.
25G knob spatula.

Dye

Triamcinolone or Trypan blue.

Tamponade

14% C_2F_6, in difficult cases 1000 cSt silicone oil.

Individual steps

1. Three-port trocar system with chandelier illumination.
2. Posterior hyaloid rhexis.
3. Posterior vitreous separation:

- Delamination of membranes with membrane pic, knob spatula and vacuum cleaner.
- Dissection of membranes with curved scissors.
- Removal of dissected membranes with vitreous cutter.

4. Hemostasis:

- Slight bleeding.
- Moderate bleeding.
- Strong bleeding.

5. Endodiathermy of all breaks and injection of PFCL.
6. Removal of attached posterior hyaloid in the periphery.
7. PRP up to ora serrata.
8. Fluid against air exchange.
9. Intravitreal Avastin.
10. Postoperative tamponade.
11. Removal of trocars.

The surgery step by step: Figs. 10.1, 10.2, 10.3, 10.4, 10.5, 10.6, 10.7, 10.8, 10.9, 10.10, 10.11, 10.12, 10.13, 10.14, 10.15 and 10.16.

1. Three-port trocar system with chandelier illumination
Insert first three trocars and then inferonasally the chandelier light. Continue with a core vitrectomy. We recommend 27G trocars (Fig. 10.1), an alternative is a hybrid system.

Surgical pearls number 102
Corneal lubrication: A major problem during vitrectomy, especially in combined surgeries with a duration of over 1 hour, is corneal epithelial edema. With the application of methylcellulose (Celoftal®, Alcon or Ocucoat®, Bausch & Lomb)

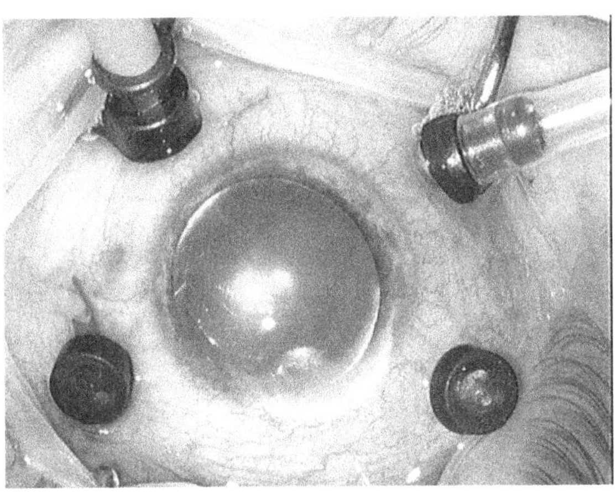

Fig. 10.1 A three-port vitrectomy with chandelier light is the best surgical setup for a difficult PDR; a chandelier light allows bimanual surgery and bimanual removal of membranes

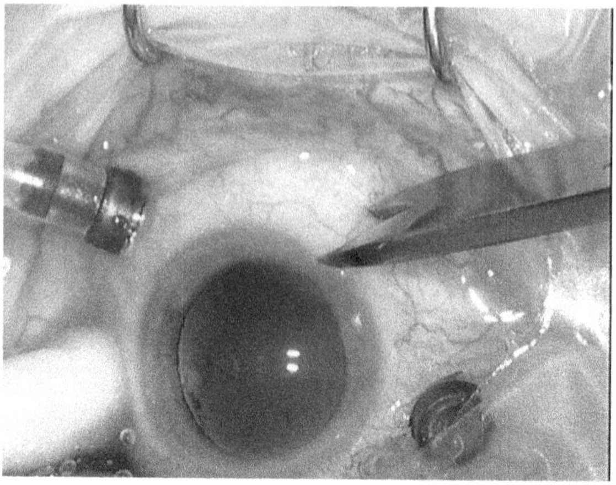

Fig. 10.2 Demonstration of the insertion of a sclera-based chandelier light (Awh, Synergetics). Rotate the globe with a cotton wool swab and mark the sclerotomy with a scleral marker

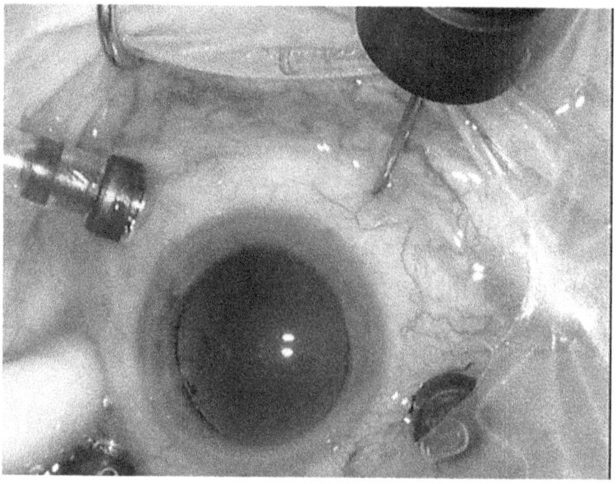

Fig. 10.3 Perform a perpendicular sclerotomy with a 25G needle from Synergetics. Use alternatively a 25G or 27G trocar stiletto knife

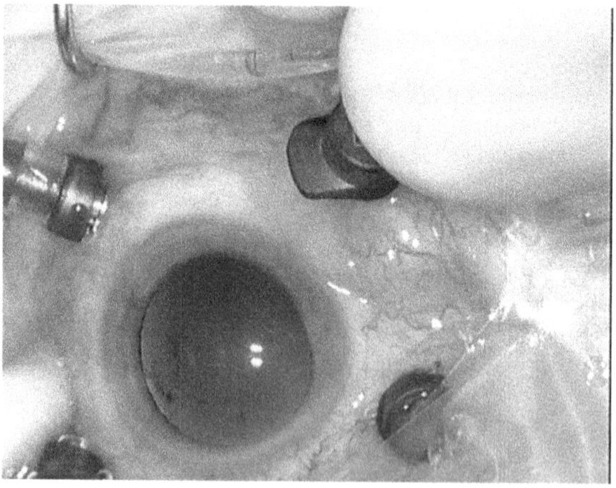

Fig. 10.4 Insert finally the chandelier light

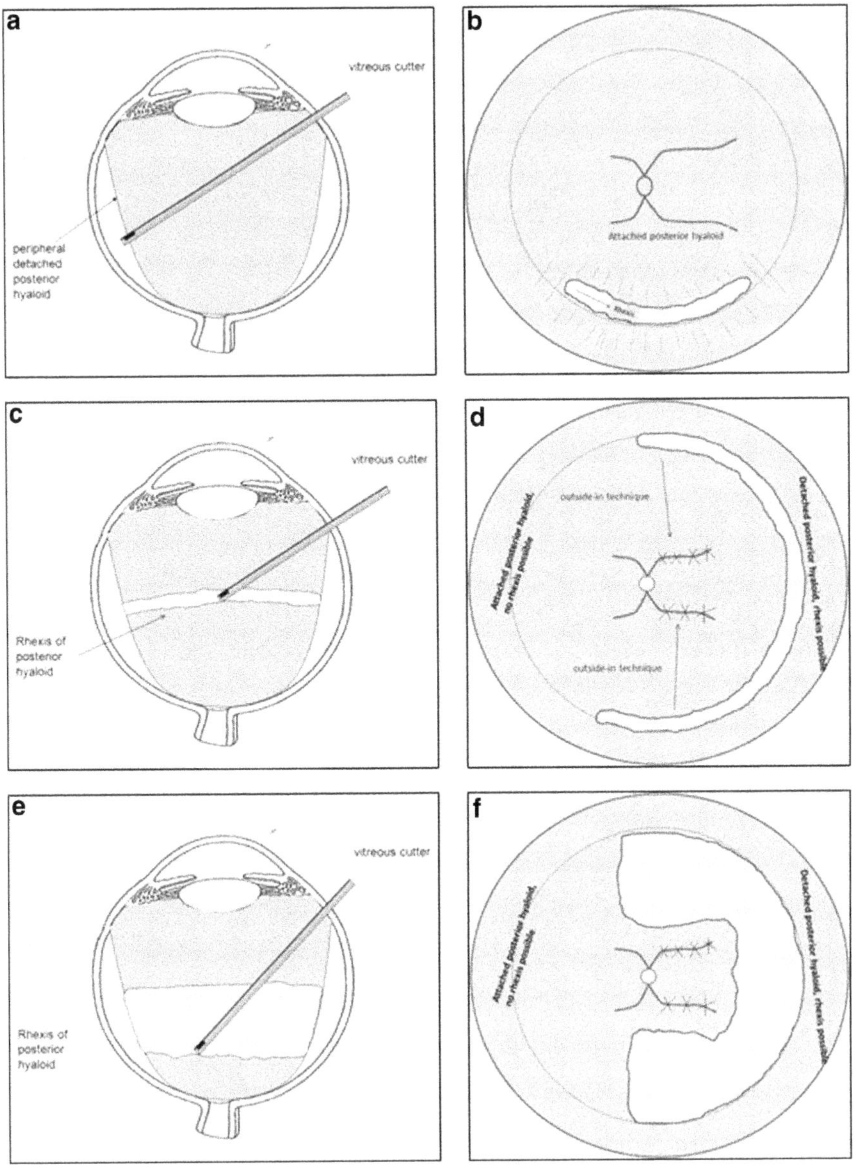

Fig. 10.5 **A–F: A/B:** The first important step of diabetic vitrectomy: The posterior hyaloid rhexis. **C/D:** Perform a rhexis of the detached posterior hyaloid on the height of the equator. **E/F:** Then continue with the removal of the vitreous to the nasal and temporal arcades. The attached (nasal) hyaloid cannot be removed in this stage (**F**)

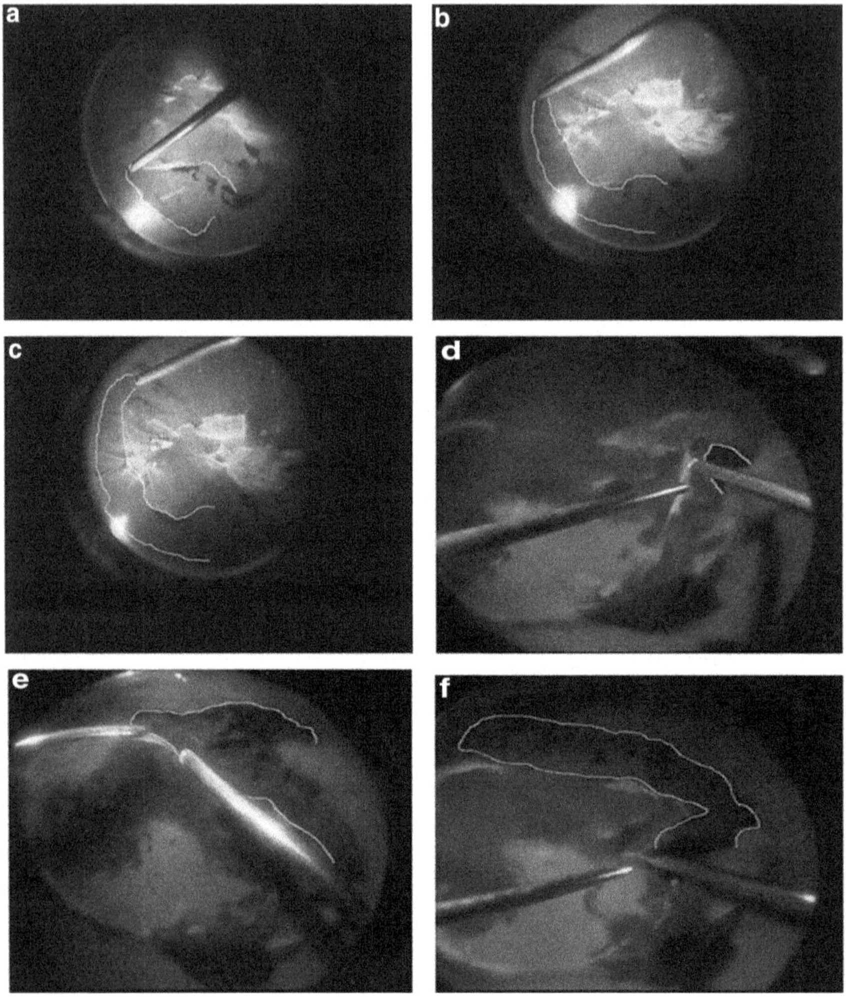

Fig. 10.6 **A–F: A:** Posterior hyaloid rhexis without subhyaloidal hemorrhage. **B:** Be careful not to damage the retina. **C:** Perform a posterior hyaloid rhexis of the detached hyaloid. A rhexis of the attached hyaloid is not possible. **D:** An opening of the posterior hyaloid with presence of subhyaloidal hemorrhage. **E:** Use the vitreous cutter with a low cutting frequency such as 1000 cuts/min. **F:** Open the posterior hyaloid as far as possible, i.e. try to perform a round rhexis as far as possible

on the cornea, the cornea can remain clear for many hours. A debridement of the epithelium is rarely necessary, but if needed use a broad blade (crescent knife).

The scleral fixated chandelier light from Synergetics is trickier to be put in place but provides, on the other hand, an excellent panoramic illumination of the vitreous cavity. Rotate the globe with a swab in a superotemporal direction so that

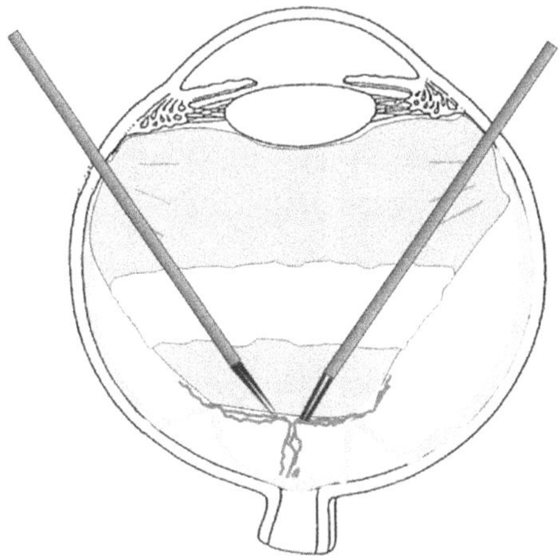

Fig. 10.7 The next and most difficult step is the bimanual removal of fibrovascular membranes

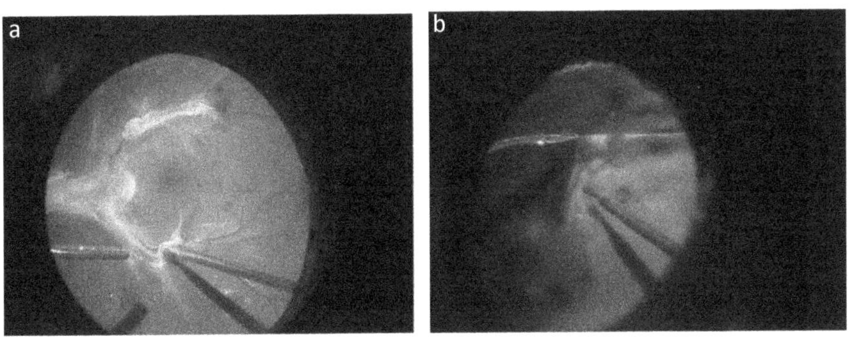

Fig. 10.8 **a** Delaminate the membrane with a knob spatula or a vacuum cleaner with silicone tip. **b** If necessary stain the posterior hyaloid with trypan blue to differentiate the membrane from the retina

there is space for the insertion of the chandelier light inferonasally. With the sclerotomy needle supplied by the manufacturer one first performs a transconjunctival sclerotomy 3.5 mm posterior to the limbus with a perpendicular (not lamellar) path. The chandelier light is then inserted into the sclerotomy. This procedure requires some practice (Figs. 10.2, 10.3 and 10.4). The Synergetics chandelier light requires an external Photon light source. An alternative is the internal light source from Constellation and EVA (requires an adapter). By bending the rigid cable of the chandelier light, you can manoeuvre the light fibre.

Surgical pearls

Insertion of a Synergetics chandelier light:

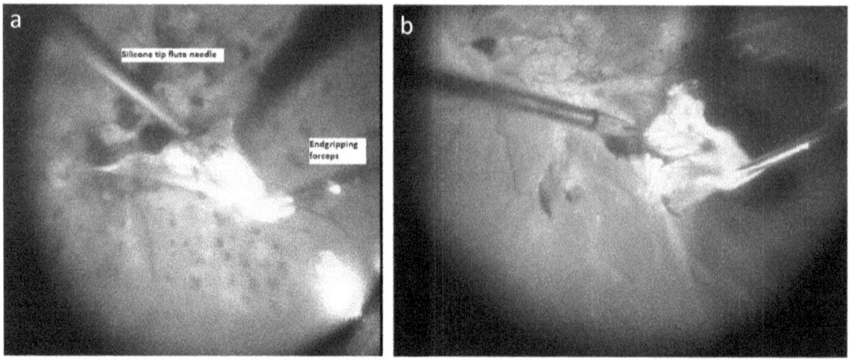

Fig. 10.9 **a** Always pull the membrane parallel to the retina. Pulling vertically may cause a choroidal bleeding or a retinal break. **b** For delamination of membranes, the knob spatula and the silicone tip flute needle are superior to the membrane pic

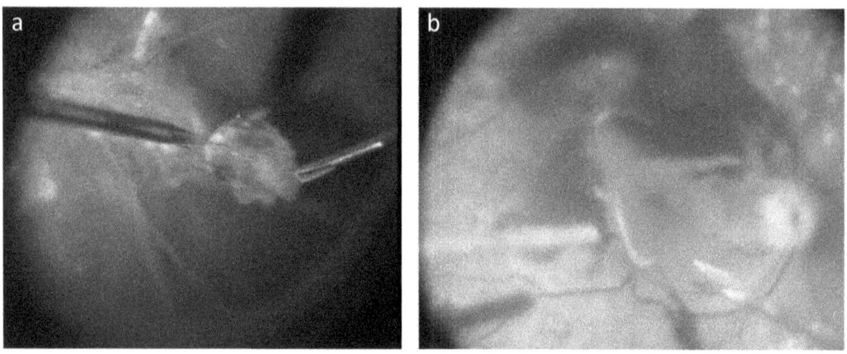

Fig. 10.10 **a** The surgeon's right hand pulls the membrane parallel to the retina and the left hand cuts the tissue bridges with the straight scissors. **b** The 27G hooked microscissors from DORC is a good alternative for cutting of vitreoretinal adhesions

(1) The insertion of the chandelier light is easier using your hands than with the trocar forceps. But you must exert a relatively strong pressure to insert the tip of the chandelier through the sclera. If you do not succeed, you can expand the sclerotomy with a 25-Gauge trocar stiletto. In case of an avitreal eye use a 23G cannula needle. The insertion is now easy, but the chandelier light sits a little loose in the sclerotomy.

(2) Conjunctival chemosis or hemorrhage may make it difficult to identify the sclerotomy. In such cases, compress the edematous conjunctiva with a normal forceps and spread the forceps tips to see the sclerotomy.

2. Posterior hyaloid rhexis (Figs. 10.5 **and** 10.6**)**

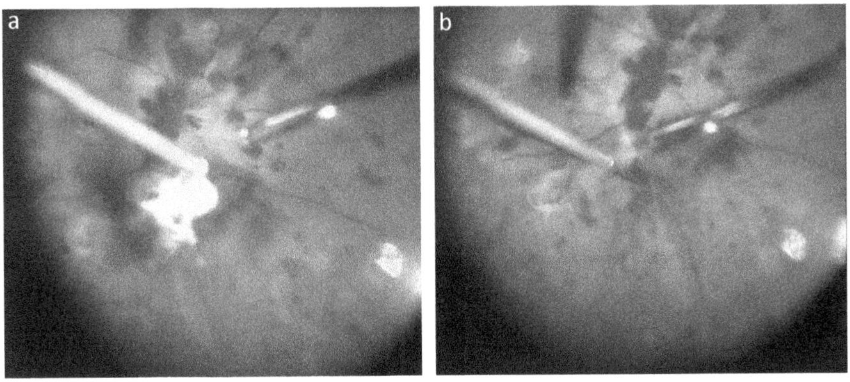

Fig. 10.11 **a** Hold the membrane in the middle of the vitreous cavity and cut the membrane. **b** The membrane is completely removed

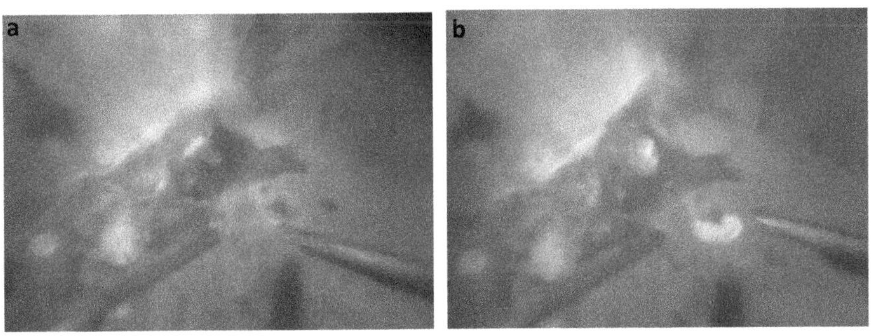

Fig. 10.12 **a** Perform a meticulous hemostasis. We use endodiathermy outside the temporal arcades and laser inside the temporal arcades. **b** Also hemostasis is performed bimanually. The surgeon's left hand holds the Charles flute needle and aspirates the blood. The right hand cauterizes the bleeding source

The posterior vitreous is usually partially detached in eyes with fibrovascular membranes. An important aim of surgery is the induction of PVD. The induction of PVD is extremely challenging in eyes with ischemic retina because the posterior hyaloid is firmly attached to the retina at many places. While trying to remove the posterior hyaloid when inducing a PVD, the surgeon can easily make tears in the ischemic thin retina.

To avoid this damage, the surgeon should begin with a peripheral vitreous detachment. In most cases of proliferative diabetic retinopathy, a partial vitreous detachment is present. This means that the vitreous is still attached centrally but partially detached in the mid-periphery. Try to find where the peripheral vitreous is detached. Create here an opening of the posterior hyaloid on the height of the equator. Then remove the vitreous along the posterior vitreous face (Figs. 10.5

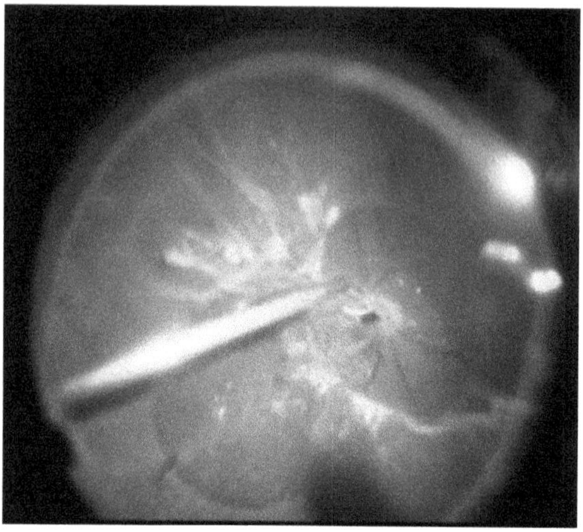

Fig. 10.13 Injection of PFCL to reattach the retina

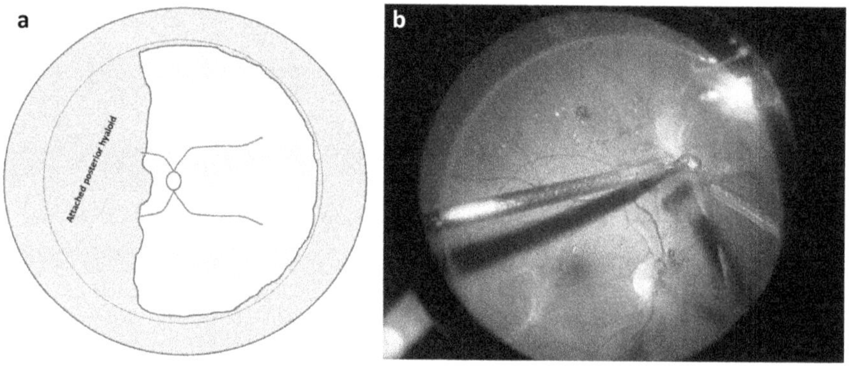

Fig. 10.14 **a** In the initial steps, a vitreous rhexis was performed and the vitreous was removed to the arcades. Then the fibrovascular membranes together with the central posterior were removed. The final step is the removal of the attached posterior hyaloid in the periphery—often on the nasal side. **b** Using a knob spatula or Charles flute needle with silicone tip the nasal pole is freed from posterior hyaloid

and 10.6) on a constant level in a circular fashion (posterior hyaloid rhexis). Do not perform a posterior hyaloid rhexis in the area where the posterior hyaloid is attached.

The surgical technique is demonstrated in these videos: 10.2 PVD_induction, 10.3 PVD_no_blood and 10.4 PVD_with_blood.

Then carefully do a vitrectomy starting from the periphery towards the beginning of the tractional membranes which are mostly near the arcades. Be careful

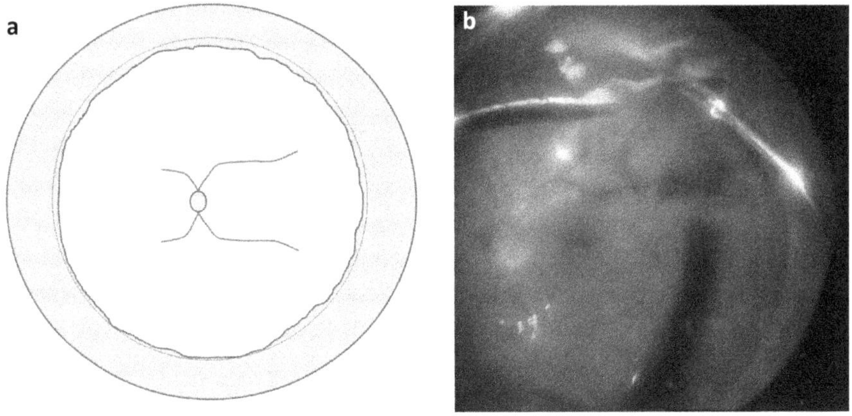

Fig. 10.15 **a** Using bimanual technique—with an endgripping forceps, knob spatula and scissors—the residual posterior hyaloid is removed up to the ora serrata. **b** Now a complete PVD has been performed. The most difficult part of the surgery has been completed

that you do not exert any pull on the membranes. If the surgeon succeeds with the posterior hyaloid rhexis, he or she can continue removing the tractional membranes bimanually.

3. Posterior vitreous separation

The fibrovascular membranes are usually located along the vascular arcades. The membranes are removed together with the posterior hyaloid. The way to success is bimanual delamination (Fig. 10.7).

For lifting the membranes, both endgripping forceps and the backflush instrument (without silicone tip) are suitable. The forceps grasp the membrane and the flute needle elevates the membrane through aspiration force.

- **Delamination of membranes with 27G Atkinson cannula and 25G vacuum cleaner or 25G knob spatula**

For delamination of the membrane, the backflush instrument with silicone tip, the 27G retrobulbar cannula (Atkinson, Beaver Visitec) and the knob spatula are suitable. We prefer the knob spatula but the backflush instrument with silicone tip and the Atkinson cannula are good alternatives. Work bimanual, with an instrument in one hand you grasp the peripheral portion of the membrane and with an instrument in the other hand you open the space between the posterior hyaloid and the underlying retina (Figs. 10.8 and 10.9). Pull the membrane always parallel to the retina. If you pull the membrane towards the lens you may create choroidal bleedings and retinal breaks. The surgical technique is shown in these videos: 10.5 Atkinson cannula, 10.6 Bimanual_peeling_with_brush_and_forceps and 10.7 Bimanual_peeling_with_knob_spatula.

- **Dissection of membranes with 27G curved or 25G straight scissors**

The membranes are partially attached by "tissue bridges" to the retina. These bridges have to be identified by careful delamination and then be cut with the straight or curved scissors (Fig. 10.10). The vertical scissors can be used for horizontal tissue bridges. The tractional membranes are dissected and removed through a constant change of instruments between delamination and cauterization. If a bleeding occurs during this step, then perform a hemostasis.

If you use a 27G vitreous cutter or a bevelled 25G cutter you can cut membranes. Adjust your settings to 400–500 cuts/min and 200–300 mmHg aspiration. Be cautious to elevate the membrane before you cut in order to avoid a retinal damage. If you are in the right plane the membrane dissection proceeds smoothly and easily. In many cases of diabetic vitrectomy, there will be vitreoschisis, so stain and see in case of a difficult membrane peeling. If you are leaving a vitreous sheet beneath proceed to the actual plane which lies beneath and restart peeling. The surgical technique is demonstrated in these videos: 10.8 Bimanual_peeling_with_scissors_1 and 10.9 Bimanual peeling with scissors_2.

- **Removal of dissected membranes with vitreous cutter**

Grasp the already dissected membrane with intravitreal forceps and hold it in the middle of the vitreous cavity. Then cut it with the vitreous cutter (1000–2000 cuts/min) (Fig. 10.11). The surgical technique can be seen in this video: 9.10 Bimanual_peeling_with_cutter.

Surgical pearls

<u>Peeling and choroidal hemorrhage:</u> Do not pull a membrane forward to the lens—you may cause a choroidal hemorrhage or a retinal break. Pull the membrane parallel to the retina.

4. Hemostasis

There are different methods to stop intraoperative bleeding, depending on its severity:

- **Slight bleeding:**

Increase the intraocular pressure to approximately 40 mmHg, aspirate the blood with the left hand and cauterize the bleeding source with endodiathermy or the laser probe in the right hand. Inside the arcades, we cauterize the bleeding sites with laser. Outside the arcades, we cauterize retinal bleeding sites with endodiathermy (Fig. 10.12). Start with relatively low energy, as too vigorous endodiathermy may create breaks in ischemic retinal tissue. Avoid diathermy on the disc; this may cause destruction of nerve fibre bundles. If the bleeding occurs within the temporal vascular arcades, then use a laser probe to cauterize the bleeding instead. Often you have to work bimanually.

- **Moderate bleeding of retina and optic disc:**

In the case of a strong bleeding source, gently press the knob spatula or the vitreous cutter for about 1 minute over the bleeding source (1 minute is longer than most people think).

- **Severe bleeding:**

If the bleeding is so severe that there is no view of the fundus, and despite aspiration with the flute needle it does not clear up, then you should perform a fluid x air exchange. The bleeding will stop. Now try to cauterize the bleeding source with endodiathermy or compress it mechanically with the knob spatula. The vitrectomy can also be continued in an air-filled vitreous cavity. Another alternative is silicone oil. One can either work under silicone oil or end surgery with a silicone oil tamponade with Avastin. The surgical technique can be viewed in these videos: 10.11 Hemostasis and 10.12 Hemostasis with knob spatula.

Surgical pearls
Intraoperative hemorrhage and adrenaline: If there is constant bleeding from several vessels under surgery then add adrenaline to the BSS bottle. Adrenaline will constrict the vessels and reduce the bleeding. Use adrenaline with caution as mentioned before.

5. Endodiathermy of all breaks and injection of PFCL
Mark meticulously all breaks with endodiathermy. If the central pole is detached then inject PFCL (Fig. 10.13) up to the equator. The presence of PFCL facilitates the removal of membranes in the periphery. After removal of all membranes inject up to the ora serrata. PRP is also performed under PFCL.

6. Removal of attached posterior hyaloid in the periphery
Trim the peripheral vitreous and the vitreous base with a bimanual technique. Indent the sclera with the sclera depressor and cut the vitreous with the vitreous cutter.

After removal of the posterior hyaloid from the posterior pole, remove the residual attached posterior hyaloid in the periphery. Remember: the posterior hyaloid in the periphery in most cases is only partially detached. The detached part with a posterior hyaloid rhexis was opened in the beginning. Now the attached part (usually nasal) must be removed. This part is firmly attached to the retina (Fig. 10.14). Simply inducing a PVD with the vitreous cutter does not work because this creates retinal tears. The surgeon must delaminate the posterior hyaloid with a bimanual technique. The posterior hyaloid has to be removed up to the vitreous base (Fig. 10.15).

Surgical pearls:
The posterior hyaloid has to be removed up to the vitreous base.

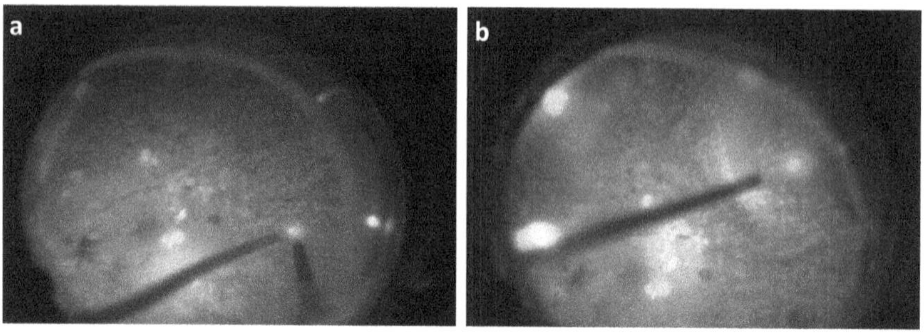

Fig. 10.16 **a** Perform a dense PRP from the arcades to the ora serrata. **b** Use preferably a curved laser probe for better access in order to perform a laser treatment up to the ora serrata

7. Panretinal photocoagulation (PRP) up to ora serrata BSS (Fig. 10.16)

The next step is a PRP. Perform a dense PRP from the arcades up to the ora serrata. By using the scleral depressor, the surgeon can laser treat up to the ora serrata.

After endolaser photocoagulation check if a new hemorrhage has occurred at the central pole and treat it before moving on to the tamponade. The surgical technique can be viewed in this video: 9.13 PFCL_Laser.

Surgical pearls

Postoperative vitreous hemorrhages are the number one problem following vitrectomy for proliferative diabetic retinopathy. In order to lower the rate of this complication, be meticulous with hemostasis. Watch out for small oozing bleeding sites after PRP has been performed. Even small collections of blood point at continuous bleeding sites that should be treated before closing up.

8. Fluid against air exchange (Fig. 10.17)

Perform a fluid against air exchange. In case of 25G or 27G, use active aspiration with backflush instrument or use the vitreous cutter. The surgical technique can be viewed in this video: 10.14 Tamponade_Air.

Air bubbles behind IOL: During a fluid-air exchange, the water condenses at the posterior surface of the IOL in the area of the capsulotomy, thereby greatly impairing the view of the fundus. It can be removed either with a flute instrument or injection of viscoelastics onto the posterior surface of the IOL.

9. Intravitreal Avastin

Inject 0.1 ml Avastin intravitreal at the end of surgery.

10. Postoperative tamponade

In young type 1 diabetics, we prefer 20% SF6 or 14% C_2F_6 as postoperative tamponade because it causes less postoperative secondary glaucoma compared to silicone oil. Silicone oil may result in secondary glaucoma after silicone oil removal. We use silicone oil in difficult cases, extensive retinal bleeding and in

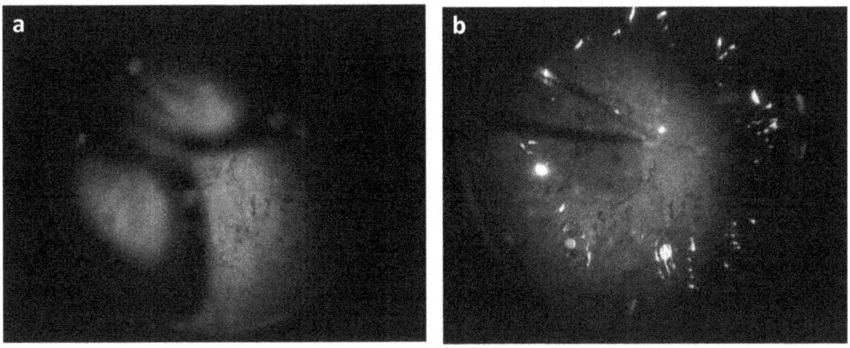

Fig. 10.17 **a** We perform in almost all cases a fluid against air exchange. If the vitreous cavity is filled with PFCL we perform a PFCL against air exchange and then the tamponade. In this case with a detached retina we would use 1000 cSt silicone oil. **b** For 23G we use a Charles flute needle with passive aspiration. For 25G and 27G, we use Charles flute needle with active aspiration

functionally only eyed patients. In old type 2 diabetics, we use in the most cases only an air tamponade. The surgical technique can be viewed in this video: 10.15 Tamponade_Silicone.

Surgical pearls:
Gas or silicone oil tamponade. If you are a beginner choose silicone oil. If you are experienced try to switch to gas.

Surgical pearls
Lens-sparing vitrectomy: In young diabetic patients, we experienced good results with a lens-sparing vitrectomy and then a C_2F_6 gas or 1000 cSt silicone oil tamponade. Even after 10–20 years the lens hardly opacifies.

10. Removal of trocars
If silicone oil is used, one should suture the sclerotomies, otherwise oil might flow under the conjunctiva. Suture 25G sclerotomies with Vicryl 8–0. 27G sclerotomies require usually no suture.

10.4 Complications

(1) Injury of a retinal artery during peeling. A fibrovascular membrane may obscure the temporal arcade. Be careful with delamination here. Begin with blunt instruments such as a knob spatula or a vacuum cleaner. Be careful when using scissors. Prefer a curved scissors as the blades conform to the curvature of the globe (27G curved scissors, DORC).
(2) Extensive bleeding: (1) Increase IOP to 60mmHG and cauterize the bleeding vessel. (2) Gently press the tip of the vitreous cutter or the knob spatula onto

the bleeding vessel for 1 minute. (3) Perform a BSS against air exchange and try to cauterize the vessel. (4) Inject silicone oil and anti-VEGF and close the case; reoperate when the bleeding has subsided.

10.5 FAQ

Which type of silicone oil you use?
We use routinely 1000/1300 cSt silicone oil. We remove the oil after 3 months. We see no advantage of using 5000 cSt oil in diabetic cases, even with tractional detachment.

What procedure do you recommend in case of an eye with iris rubeosis, cataract and vitreous hemorrhage?
Do not operate this eye before the iris rubeosis is treated and has disappeared. We would inject immediately 0.1 ml Avastin. After 1 month, we would perform a combined phacoemulsification + IOL implantation + intravitreal 0.1 ml Avastin. Again 1 month later we would perform a vitrectomy.

What procedure do you recommend in case of an old type 2 diabetic with vitreous hemorrhage secondary to diabetes?
I would schedule a phaco + Avastin. One month later I would perform a vitrectomy with laser, Avastin and air tamponade.

What type of gas do you use?
We use routinely air for easy cases and 20% Sf_6 and 14% C_2F_6 for difficult cases.

Is it necessary to remove all membranes?
Remove all membranes with a tractional component. You can leave membranes without a tractional component.

If you do not have the required instruments or experience to remove all membranes then don't do it. You will cause more harm than good. Remove instead the posterior hyaloid from the periphery to the posterior pole so that the tractions can relax, then perform a scatter laser and stop surgery. The surgery will reduce the tractional detachment and maybe sufficient.

Three complete surgeries can be viewed in these videos:

Chapter 10: A total retinal detachment secondary to diabetes, https://youtu.be/UNaRKZhByPo.

Chapter 10: Advanced TRD for diabetic retinopathy, https://youtu.be/qLUpRXD1CJ4.

Chapter 10: Advanced proliferative diabetic retinopathy with detachment of posterior pole, https://youtu.be/yvBtGct61uA.

11 Surgery of Laser Untreated Difficult Diabetic Vitrectomy

The typical patient is young type I diabetic patient with poor compliance. All screening appointments have been missed and no laser or anti-VEGF treatment has been performed. Both eyes have a PDR with tractional retinal detachment, in one eye the macula is detached and in the fellow eye the VA has recently decreased. The main features of advanced PDR with TRD are

TRD.

not laser treated (no PRP).

no PVD.

Many VR surgeons perform an immediate vitrectomy. We recommend to avoid an immediate vitrectomy because the risk for surgical failure in these eyes is especially high. We recommend instead an immediate pretreatment with anti-VEGF and laser and a delayed vitrectomy.

Our treatment planning is shown in Fig. 11.1. We perform an immediate anti-VEGF injection to win time and start treatment. Then we plan a laser treatment in general anaesthesia. Again, 4 weeks later we perform a lens-sparing vitrectomy. *Remark*: Not pretreated means no prior laser treatment and no anti-VEGF within 3 months.

When we perform vitrectomy, the membranes are dry and avascular. Endodiathermy is not required so that you can concentrate fully on the removal of the tractional posterior vitreous. The surgical management of this vitrectomy can be found step by step in the chapter "Surgery of difficult diabetic vitrectomy".

U. Spandau and Z. Tomic, *Small-Gauge Vitrectomy for Diabetic Retinopathy*,
https://doi.org/10.1007/978-3-031-26204-3_11

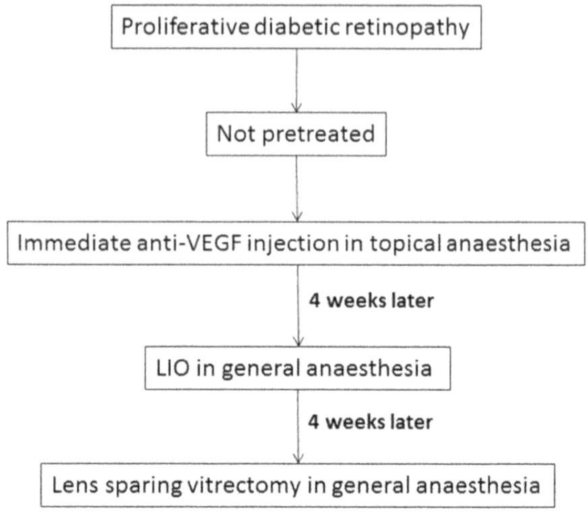

Fig. 11.1 Our treatment planning for a laser untreated difficult diabetic vitrectomy

11.1 Laser Indirect Photocoagulation of the Retina

11.1.1 Introduction

Indirect laser photocoagulation of the retina is a major tool in preventing blindness. Photocoagulation burns are applied to the ischemic retina keeping space of one burn width in between. Two laser types are used for treatment of the retina: Argon laser with a wavelength of 510 nm and diode laser with 810 nm wavelength. Argon laser has been replaced with frequency doubled Nd–Yag laser of 532 nm wavelength in most setting.

The technique of indirect laser coagulation (LIO) is difficult and requires much training. In diabetes, a laser coagulation in many sessions is possible but in case of LIO the procedure is usually done in one session.

First you must learn to examine adults with the binocular indirect ophthalmoscope. This training requires at least 3 months. Then you can start with laser coagulation. You laser one eye and your mentor lasers the fellow eye. After approximately five laser treatments with your teacher you can start to treat alone.

One eye or both eyes? This depends on the extent of the ischemia of the retina. Usually we treat both eyes.

11.1.2 Instruments for Laser Coagulation

(1) Diode laser device (Fig. 11.2).
(2) Binocular indirect ophthalmoscope (Fig. 11.3).
(3) Volk 25D lens (Fig. 11.4).
(4) Scleral depressor (Fig. 11.5).
(5) Lid speculum (Fig. 11.6).

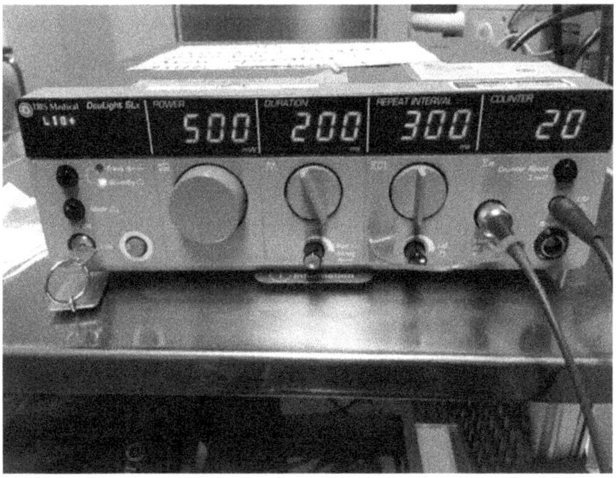

Fig. 11.2 A diode laser (Iridex) and two attached cables from binocular laser ophthalmoscope for laser and light

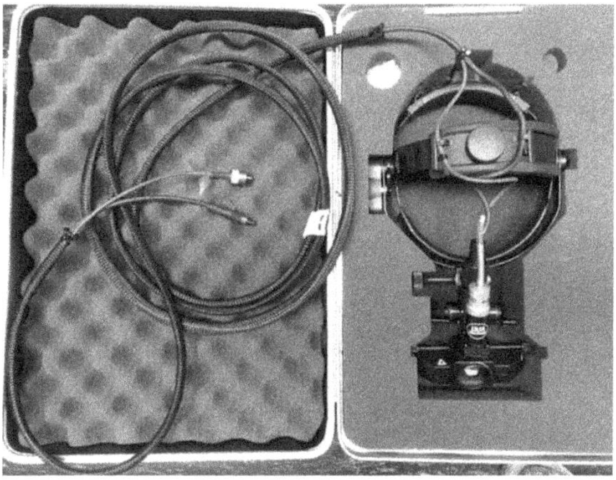

Fig. 11.3 A binocular indirect laser ophthalmoscope (LIO) (Iridex, Iridex). The two cables are attached to the laser device (Fig. 11.2)

Laser device (Fig. **11.2**)**:** We use always a diode laser (Iridex, CA). An alternative is an Argon laser. The initial settings of the laser device are 100/100/300: power: 100 mW, duration: 100 msec, interval: 300 msec.

Laser indirect ophthalmoscope (LIO) (Fig. **11.3**): The laser indirect ophthalmoscope is a helmet which contains an indirect ophthalmoscope attached to a laser device. Our laser indirect ophthalmoscope is connected to the diode laser (Iridex, CA).

Volk 25D lens (Fig. **11.4**): We use usually the 25D lens from Volk. An alternative is the 20D lens which is better for the ridge but not so good for ora serrata.

Scleral depressor (Fig. **11.5**)**:** A scleral depressor is very important for laser coagulation. You can only reach the ora serrata with a scleral depressor. If possible, we laser with the big indentor because it enables treating more tissue at once. At

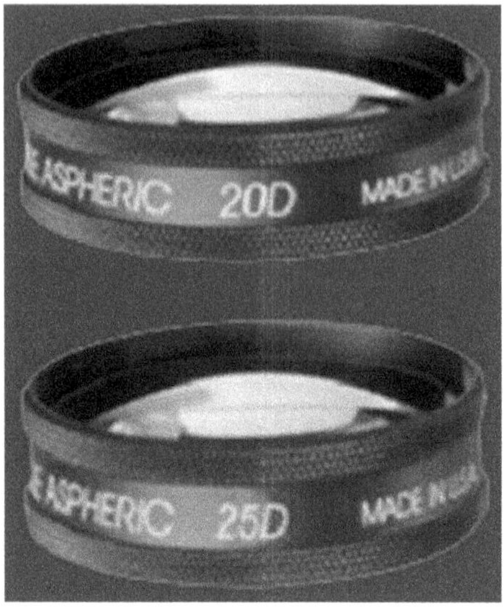

Fig. 11.4 20D and 25D lens from Volk. Both lenses are suitable for laser. We use preferably the 25D lens

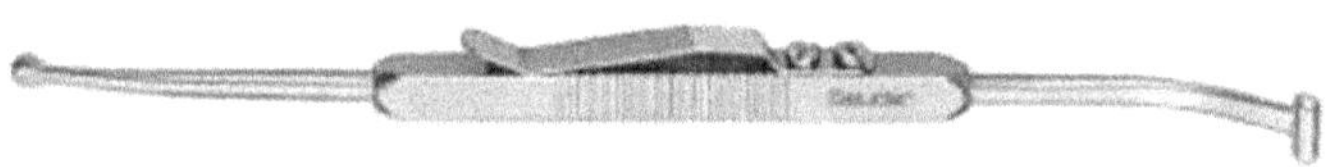

Fig. 11.5 Sclera depressor with small and large indentor (Geuder, Germany)

Fig. 11.6 Lid speculum (Geuder No. 17023, Germany)

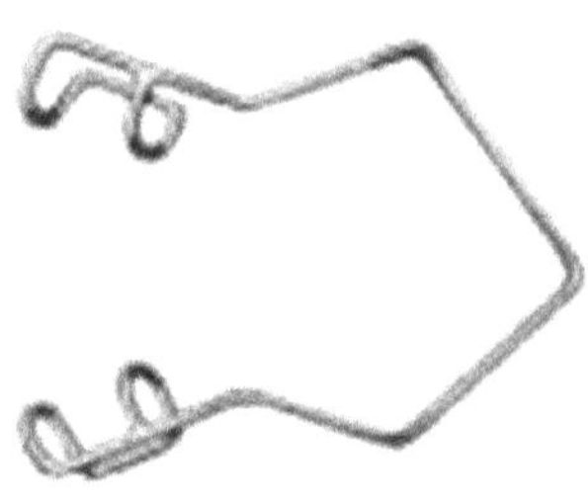

the ora serrata we prefer the small indentor. Alternatively, you can use a cotton wool swab or a Strabismus hook as an indentor.

Lid speculum (Fig. **11.6**)**:** We prefer a small lid speculum.

We use usually a diode laser. Alternatively, you can use an Argon laser. The *normal amount* of laser effects is 1200–1800 laser spots (minimum: 1000 laser spots, maximum: 2500 laser spots).

The starting settings for a diode laser are 200 mW (power), 200 ms (duration) and 300 msec (interval). Then increase the power to 400mW in stepwise manner or maybe to 450 mW. Then if required increase the duration to 250 msec and then to 300 msec.

11.1.3 Laser Treatment Step by Step

(1) Start with the temporal retina. Find the correct laser power.
(2) Laser treat the temporal retina from ora serrata almost to the ridge
(3) Laser treat the superior, nasal and inferior retina.
(4) Treat the ridge.
(5) Inspect the retina for skip lesions and incomplete laser.

The surgery in detail:
The pupil must be well dilated, a small pupil is not sufficient for laser photocoagulation. We start always with the temporal retina. Why? The temporal retina has the biggest ischemic area. Therefore, the visualization of the temporal ischemic retina is the best of all quadrants.

Indent the retina with the broad side of the sclera depressor and place a few laser spots on the indented retina (Fig. 11.7). If you do not see a laser spot, then increase power to 200 mW and try again. If you see no laser spot increase power to 300mW and continue like this until you reach 450 mW. If you still do not see a laser spot, then increase duration to 250 msec and then to 300 msec.

You should achieve a laser spot with approximately 500 mW power and 300 msec duration. If the retina bleaches very much or you see a burst in the retina with a bleeding, then the laser power is too high. Reduce power by 100 mW and try again.

Anti-VEGF injection: After laser photocoagulation we inject ant-VEGF. Anti-VEGF reduces the risk for macular edema.

Follow-up: We prescribe the eye drops Dexamethasone 1 mg/ml 2 times/d and Atropine 0.1% 2 times/d for 2 weeks.

Fig. 11.7 Start at the temporal quadrant and find the appropriate laser settings

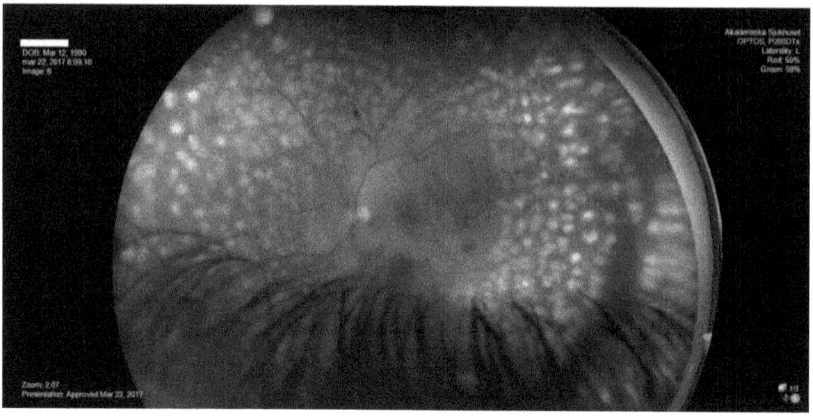

Fig. 11.8 Optos photograph, showing a 1-day postop after LIO laser treatment with 1879 spots

11.1.4 Conclusion

LIO is a medically very effective treatment. Within one session you can treat the complete eye. Laser indirect photocoagulation, however, is technically a very difficult procedure which requires much training.

11.2 Case Reports for Laser Untreated Difficult Diabetic Vitrectomy

Case 1: 19 y/o male patient with insulin-dependent diabetes and poor compliance. A PDR in both eyes was diagnosed. His eyes were not laser treated. Subsequently he was laser treated in both eyes with LIO and received an Eylea injection (Figs. 11.8 and 11.9). No vitrectomy was performed.

Case 2: A 48 y/o female patient with type 1 insulin-dependent diabetes and poor compliance. She presents with a tractional retinal detachment in her better eye. The retina is not laser treated. A laser indirect ophthalmoscopy in general anaesthesia is performed. The tractions increased after laser treatment but did not involve the macula (Fig. 11.10). One month later a vitrectomy was performed, all tractions were removed and the retina is attached without tamponade.

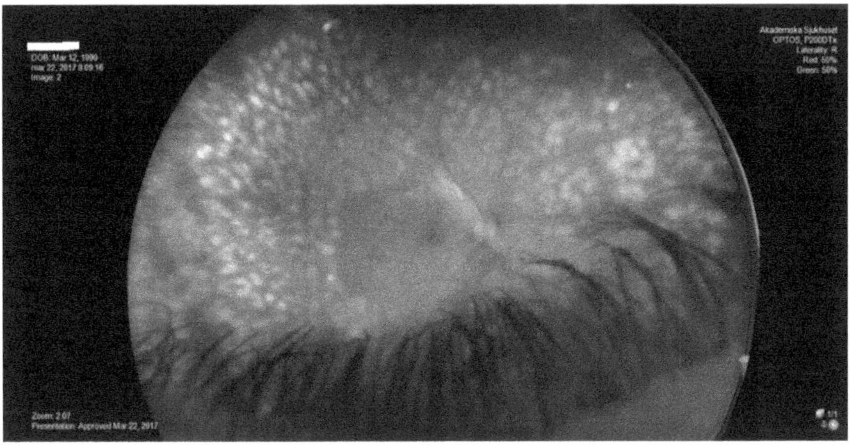

Fig. 11.9 Optos photograph, showing a 1-day postop after LIO laser treatment with 2674 spots. No vitrectomy is planned

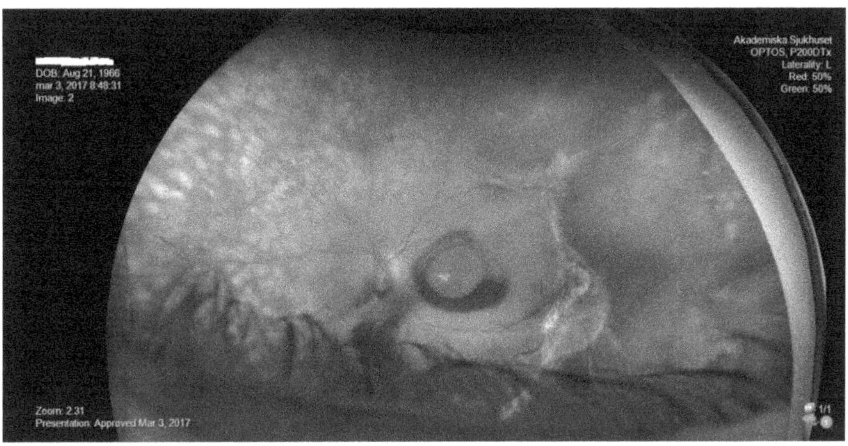

Fig. 11.10 Optos photograph showing an eye after laser treatment with 1500 laser spots. A lens-sparing vitrectomy is scheduled

Part VI

Unusual and Difficult Cases Including Neovascular Glaucoma

All videos of this book are found on the Youtube channel from Ulrich Spandau and playing list "Proliferative diabetic retinopathy" (link: https://youtube.com/playlist?list=PL0dKYclPD7yM9qRjBoF1HMwtxFfbf2T6A).

Chapter 12: Unusual and difficult cases

Chapter 12.1: https://youtu.be/FhPp4FqriI0 and https://youtu.be/BOe8bgFSlao

Chapter 12.2: https://youtu.be/c332nn-ZbV0

Chapter 12.3: https://youtu.be/vOnOfbUeuVQ

Chapter 13: Neovascular glaucoma

https://youtu.be/Dw3SvWd3X1U

12 Unusual and Difficult Cases

A vitreous hemorrhage with advanced PDR but without prior laser treatment is a surgically challenging case. A laser treatment is not possible due to the vitreous hemorrhage. We will demonstrate how to approach this case with a double vitrectomy. This technique is described in Sect. 12.1.

A completely attached posterior hyaloid with advanced PDR and retinal detachment necessitates an immediate surgery. The surgical challenge is to induce a PVD. In this case an inside-out technique can lead to surgical success. This technique is demonstrated in Sect. 12.2.

Another challenging pathology is a severe intraoperative bleeding. The latter is one of the most difficult complications in diabetic surgery. We will demonstrate how to tackle an intraoperative hemorrhage (see Sect. 12.3).

12.1 Advanced Proliferative Diabetic Retinopathy Without PVD—Double Vitrectomy

A vitreous hemorrhage with advanced PDR but without prior laser treatment is a surgically challenging case (Fig. 12.1). A laser treatment is not possible due to the vitreous hemorrhage. A PVD is not present. We will demonstrate how to operate within two sessions (double vitrectomy). Stepwise vitrectomy reduces the risk of iatrogenic retinal tears and major bleeding during surgery.

In the first vitrectomy, you start with a core vitrectomy, continue with an endolaser PRP and terminate the operation with a gas tamponade (Fig. 12.2). Then we wait 1–2 weeks and within this time a partial PVD will occur (Fig. 12.3). In the second vitrectomy, you continue by removing the fibrovascular membranes and completing the PRP (Figs. 12.4 and 12.5).

The surgical videos of this case are available under this link: Two videos are available:

https://youtu.be/FhPp4FqriI0 and https://youtu.be/BOe8bgFSlao

U. Spandau and Z. Tomic, *Small-Gauge Vitrectomy for Diabetic Retinopathy*,
https://doi.org/10.1007/978-3-031-26204-3_12

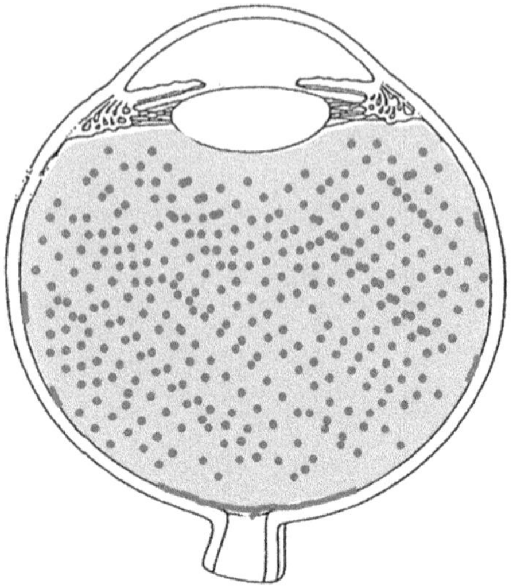

Fig. 12.1 **Second method:** Advanced PDR with vitreous hemorrhage. The eye has never been laser treated. A laser treatment is not possible because of vitreous hemorrhage. Note that the posterior vitreous is attached

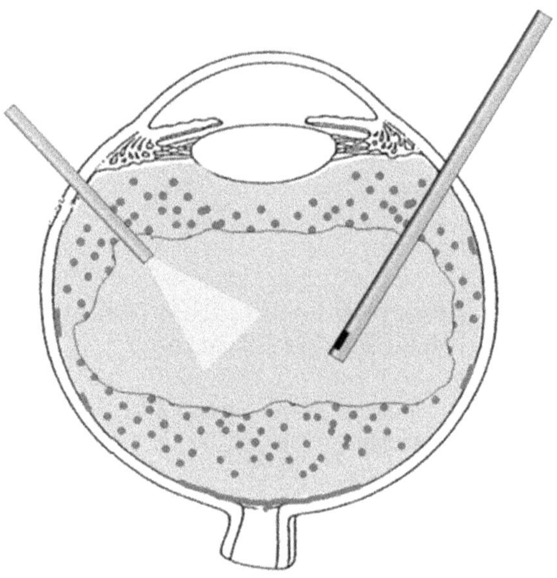

Fig. 12.2 A core vitrectomy is performed and then a dense PRP up to the ora serrata is performed. After a gas tamponade, the operation is finished. No membrane peeling is performed

First vitrectomy:

1. **3-port vitrectomy with/without chandelier illumination**
2. **Core vitrectomy**
3. **PRP**
4. **Gas tamponade and anti-VEGF**

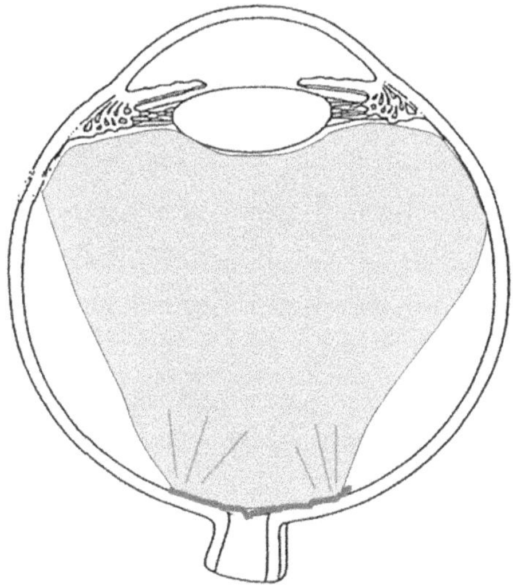

Fig. 12.3 During the following week a (spontaneous) peripheral PVD will occur. The peripheral retina is attached

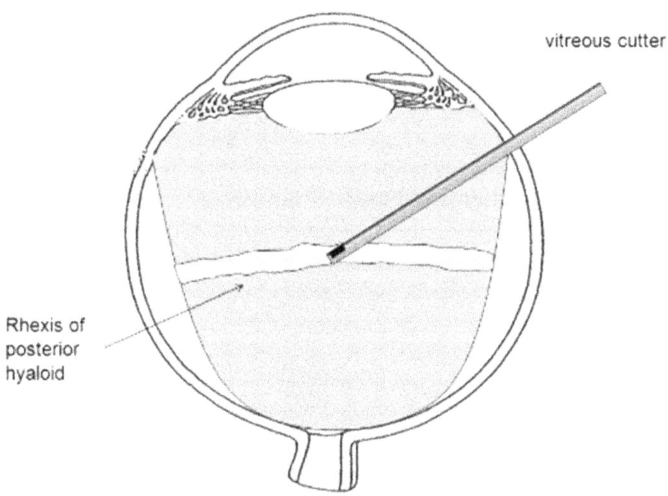

Fig. 12.4 Now, we have a situation as we like it. A peripheral PVD is present. The second surgery can be scheduled. Perform a posterior hyaloid rhexis

Perform a core vitrectomy. If the posterior hyaloid is attached, continue with PRP. If a subhyaloidal hemorrhage is present, then perform a posterior hyaloid rhexis, aspirate the subhyaloidal blood and perform a PRP. End the surgery with a 20% SF_6 tamponade and an anti-VEGF injection.

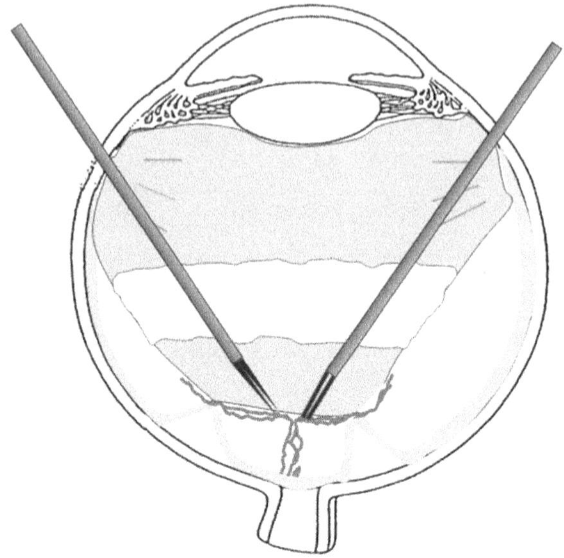

Fig. 12.5 Continue then with a bimanual removal of the fibrovascular membranes

Second vitrectomy:

1. **3-port vitrectomy with chandelier illumination**
2. **Posterior hyaloid rhexis**
3. **Removal of membranes**
4. **Hemostasis**
5. **Vitreous base shaving**
6. **(Silicone oil) tamponade and anti-VEGF**

In the second surgery the preretinal membranes are removed. Insert a chandelier light to enable a bimanual removal. After removal of the membranes, a fill-in PRP is performed and a 1000 cSt silicone oil tamponade is performed.

Comment to stepwise surgery: In principle, one should perform stepwise surgery in every case with advanced PDR without PRP and without PVD; if there are broad or ill-defined connections between proliferations and the retina (cleavage) and/or active proliferations with broad and pronounced vascular invasion. With stepwise surgery in such cases you reduce the risk of iatrogenic retinal holes and major bleeding during surgery. Stepwise surgery is impossible if there is already TRD with macular engagement, which usually contains a rhegmatogenous component (TRD + RRD). In such a case, you lose more if you do not reattach the macula directly.

Conclusion: The aim of the first vitrectomy is to convert an attached vitreous to a partial PVD and to reduce the vascular activity of the retina. The aim of the second vitrectomy is to induce a complete PVD.

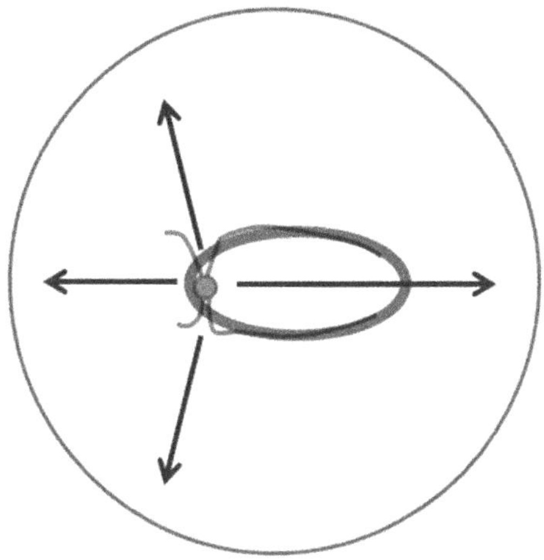

Fig. 12.6 Inside-out technique. The membranes are removed from the posterior pole to the periphery. This is not the normal technique for diabetic vitrectomy

12.2 Membrane Removal with Disc to Periphery Technique

The correct surgical technique for membrane removal for diabetic retinopathy is the outside-in (periphery to disc) technique. In contrast, the disc to periphery (in-outside) technique is atypical for diabetic vitrectomy. The latter technique is necessary if the posterior hyaloid is completely attached. You start to induce a central PVD and work your way towards the ora serrata (Fig. 12.6).

Case report: A 43 y/o male patient with diabetes mellitus type 1 was admitted to the clinic for the treatment of advanced PDR with TRD and rhegmatogenous retinal detachment in his RE. He was treated before with incomplete laser PRP in both eyes. The visual acuity in the right eye was CF at 2 m and in left eye CF at 3 m.

He underwent a combined phaco/vitrectomy with en-bloc excision of all visible proliferations, endodrainage of subretinal fluid through the existing retinal tear, completed with extended endolaser PRP up to ora serrata and silicone oil 1300 cSt tamponade (Figs. 12.7, 12.8, 12.9, 12.10, 12.11, 12.12, 12.13, 12.14, 12.15 and 12.16). The post operative visual acuity in the RE two months after surgery was 0.1 and the retina was completely attached. The patient is scheduled for a silicone oil removal in a month.

The surgical video of this case is available under this link: https://youtu.be/FhPp4FqriI0.

12.3 Severe Intraoperative Bleeding, "The Bloody Eye"

Extensively bleeding fibrovascular membranes are the most difficult and challenging surgical complication in ocular surgery because you simply do not see what you are doing. Intraoperative bleeding is quite common during diabetic surgery. Fortunately, in most cases, the bleeding can be easily controlled. The best option

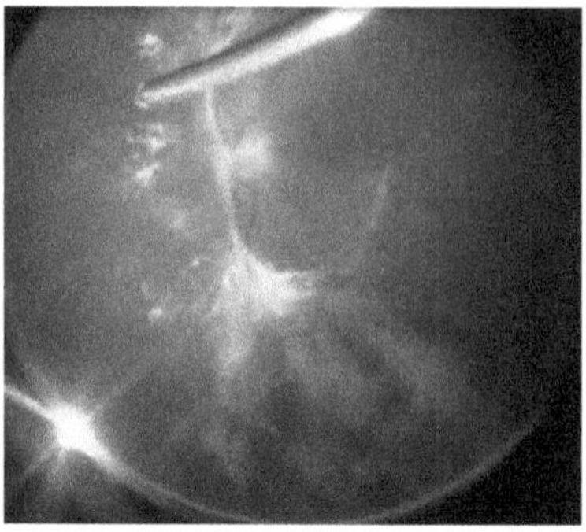

Fig. 12.7 An advanced PDR with attached posterior hyaloid and no laser treatment

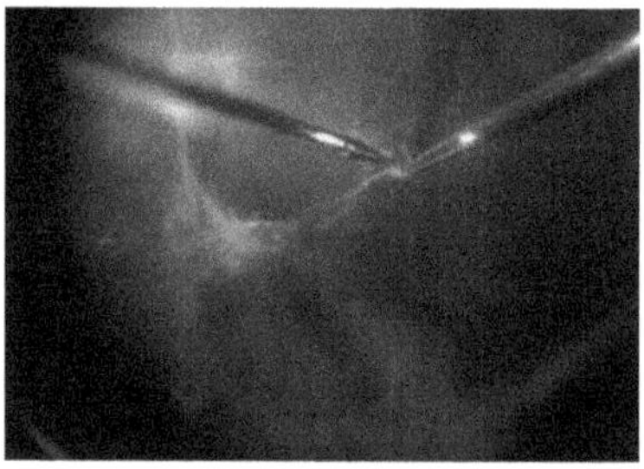

Fig. 12.8 Attempt to open the posterior hyaloid at the posterior pole with a disc to periphery technique

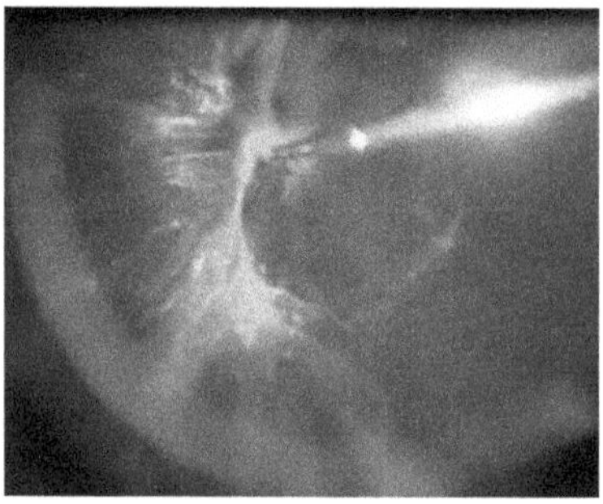

Fig. 12.9 Opening of posterior hyaloid at the optic disc

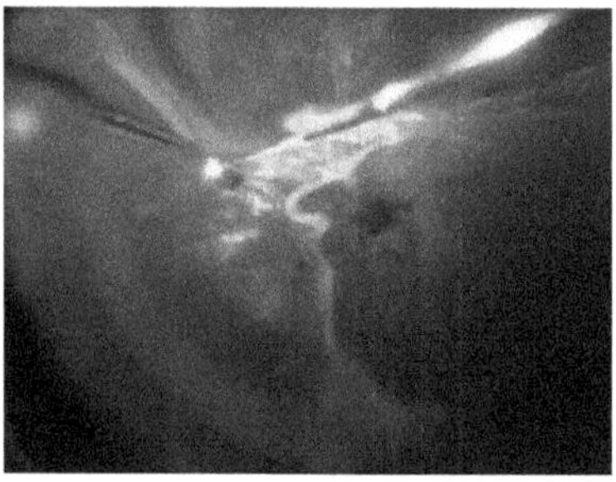

Fig. 12.10 The central part of the posterior hyaloid is delaminated

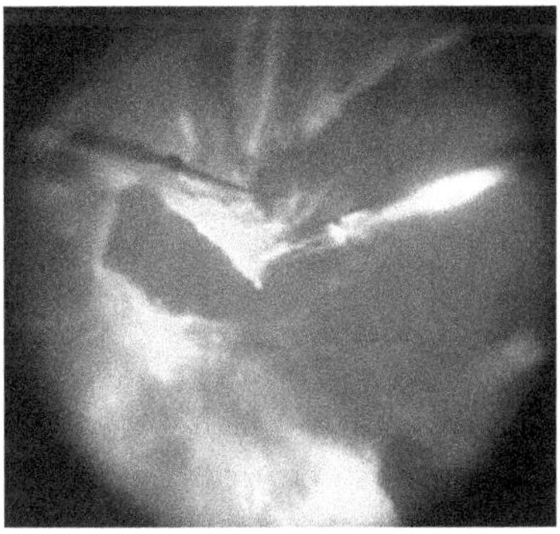

Fig. 12.11 Delamination of posterior hyaloid at the superior retina

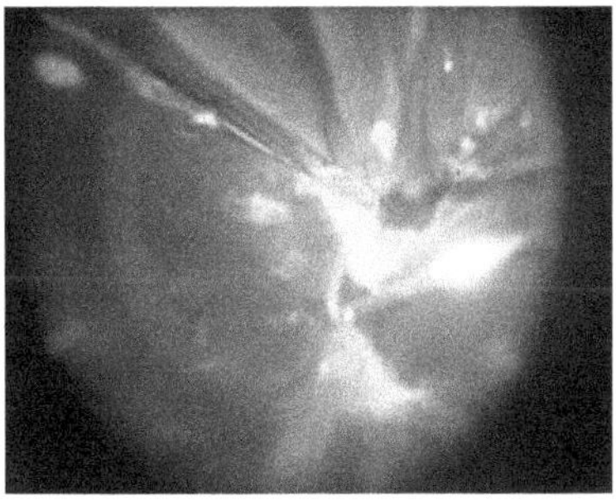

Fig. 12.12 The bimanual delamination is performed with straight scissors (left) and intravitreal forceps (right)

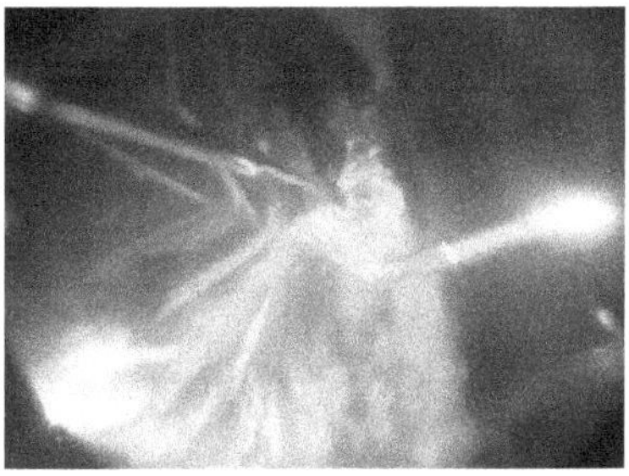

Fig. 12.13 The posterior hyaloid must be removed up to the vitreous base

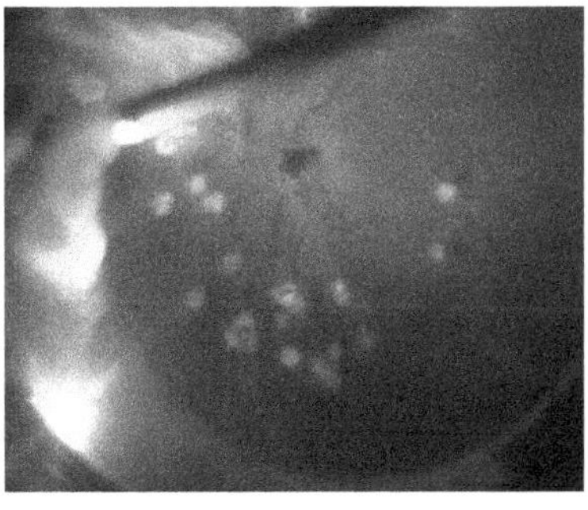

Fig. 12.14 Vitreous base shaving. Note the endodiathermy effects in the retina

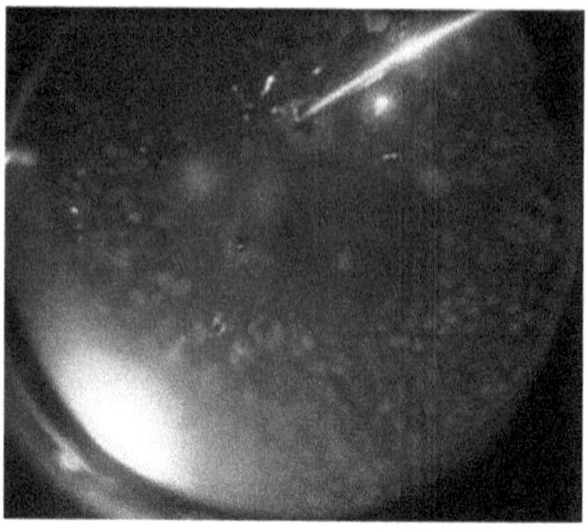

Fig. 12.15 An air-filled vitreous cavity. A PRP up to the ora serrata is performed

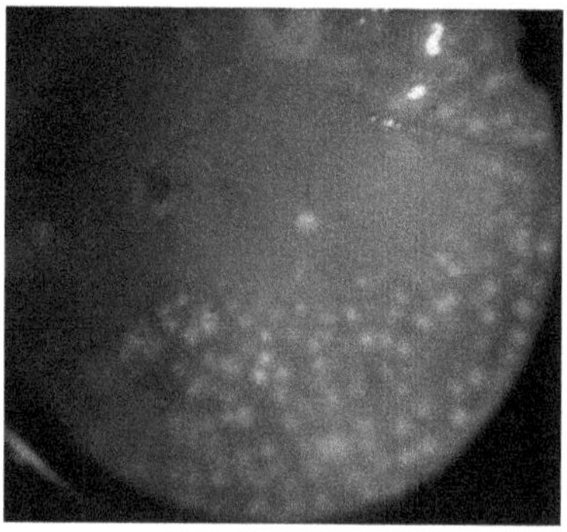

Fig. 12.16 Finally 1300 cSt silicone oil is injected

is to perform a PRP, terminate the operation and reoperate after 4 weeks. If you decide to continue then employ the following surgical options. The surgical video of this case is available under this link:

https://youtu.be/ry9NNC0t33w

Following countermeasures can be applied:

(1) Aggressive endodiathermy
(2) Fluid against air exchange and peeling under air
(3) Injection of silicone oil and peeling under silicone oil
(4) Injection of silicone oil and Avastin and terminate the operation

(1) Aggressive endodiathermy

As long as you work outside the temporal arcades you can and should use aggressively endodiathermy. Start peeling at one location and switch between delamination of the membrane and endodiathermy of bleeding sources (Fig. 12.17). Do not continue with peeling until the peeled retina is dry.

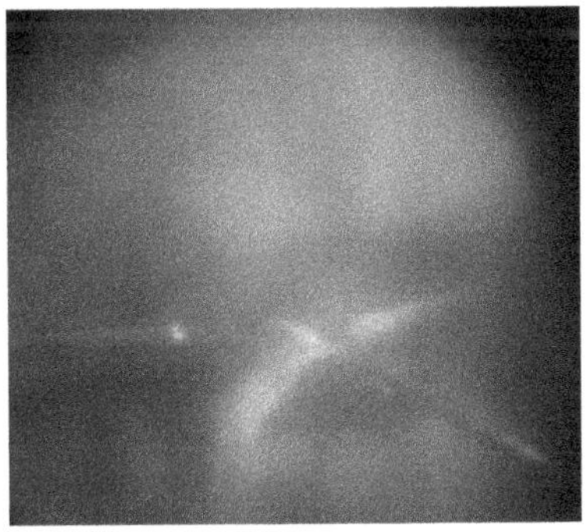

Fig. 12.17 Peeling under BSS. Peeling of fibrovascular membranes under poor visibility secondary to vitreous hemorrhage

(2) Fluid against air exchange and peeling under air

If you have no view of the retina due to excessive blood in the vitreous cavity, then perform a fluid against air exchange. Try to identify the bleeding source and cauterize the bleeding source. You can even remove vitreous body under air and partially membranes (Fig. 12.18).

(3) Injection of silicone oil and peeling under silicone oil

An alternative to an air tamponade is a silicone oil tamponade. The huge advantage of silicone oil is the good view. You can even continue to peel the membranes (Fig. 12.19), a vitrectomy is however not possible.

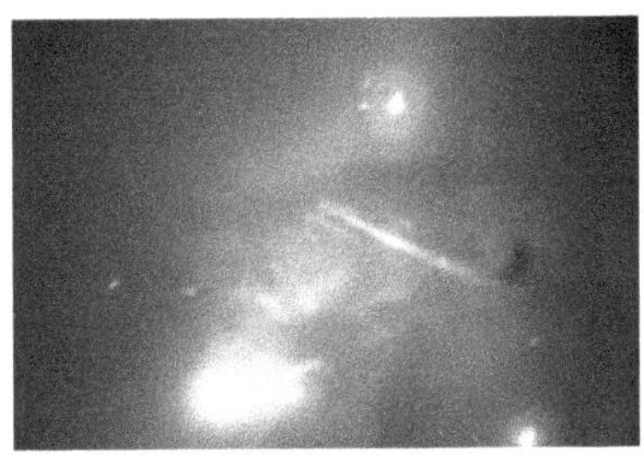

Fig. 12.18 Peeling under air. The same eye with improved visibility due to air in the vitreous cavity. The peeling is however more difficult because the air presses the tissue against the retina

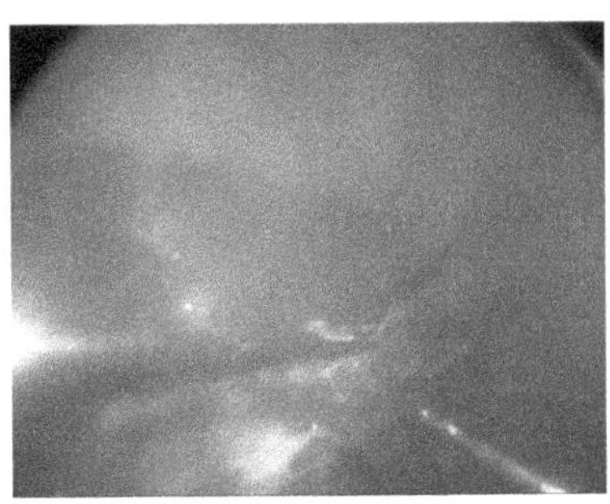

Fig. 12.19 Peeling under silicone oil. The best visibility of all tamponades. The peeling is easier because silicone oil presses the membranes with less force against the retina. Remember: Surface tension of silicone oil is less than air

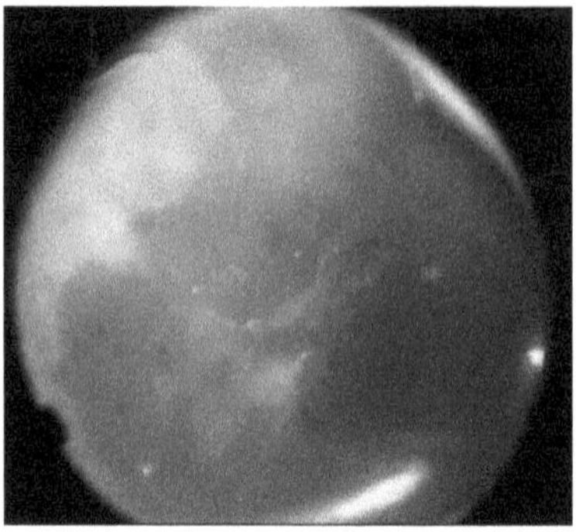

Fig. 12.20 It is therefore a very good option to inject silicone oil and Avastin and wait 1–4 weeks for the next surgery

PFCL is not such a good alternative because the blood in the vitreous cavity settles on the apex of the PFCL bubble which is not the case for silicone oil. You can remove the blood but it easily reoccurs.

(4) Injection of silicone oil and Avastin and terminate the operation

If the bleeding is too excessive and you cannot localize the bleeding source, then don't hesitate to terminate the operation. In order to improve the conditions for the next surgery, inject silicone oil and inject Avastin (Fig. 12.20). If the hemorrhage has subsided during follow-up, after approximately four weeks, schedule the final surgery.

Neovascular Glaucoma 13

The most common indication for neovascular glaucoma in our country is an ischemic CRVO. The most patients have light perception, a few cases have a useful vision. We inform the patients that the vision does not improve after therapy and that the aim of surgery is to prevent a deterioration of vision and the preservation of the eye.

We perform a retinal cryopexy under BIOM view. The big advantage of this technique is that you see the retina and the bleaching of the cryopexy effects. Even if the cornea is edematous you have a sufficient view to the retina. We perform a 360° limbal peritomy because a cryopexy damages the goblet cells and induces a significant conjunctival chemosis. A retrobulbar anaesthesia is required. Prescribe pain medication for 2 postoperative weeks because this surgery causes significant postoperative pain. Be cautious with cryopexy of ciliary body because the eye can terminate in a hypotony. The link for this surgery is https://youtu.be/Dw3SvWd3X1U.

13.1 Treatment Planning for Neovascular Glaucoma

We treat neovascular glaucoma first with an intravitreal anti-VEGF injection and wait for 4 weeks. See treatment planning in Fig. 13.1. What is the advantage of this stepwise procedure? The neovascular stimulus and the IOP decrease significantly after 4 weeks, several patients do not wish a further treatment. We inform, however, our patients that the iris rubeosis will recur if a cryopexy is not performed.

An injection of 0.05 anti-VEGF solution into an eye with high IOP is no problem. We perform injections in eyes with IOP of 54 mmHg without any problem. We do not perform an AC tap. *Remark*: Be careful with an injection in a small eye (microphthalmia). To avoid an excessive IOP increase, give the patient 500 mg acetazolomide 2 hours before injection.

U. Spandau and Z. Tomic, *Small-Gauge Vitrectomy for Diabetic Retinopathy*,
https://doi.org/10.1007/978-3-031-26204-3_13

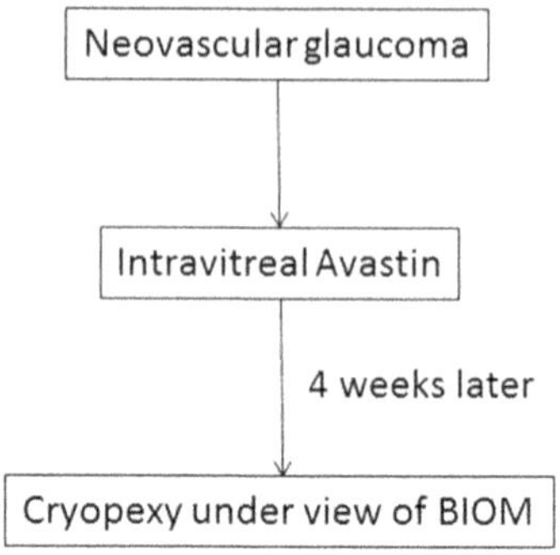

Fig. 13.1 Treatment planning for neovascular glaucoma at our hospital

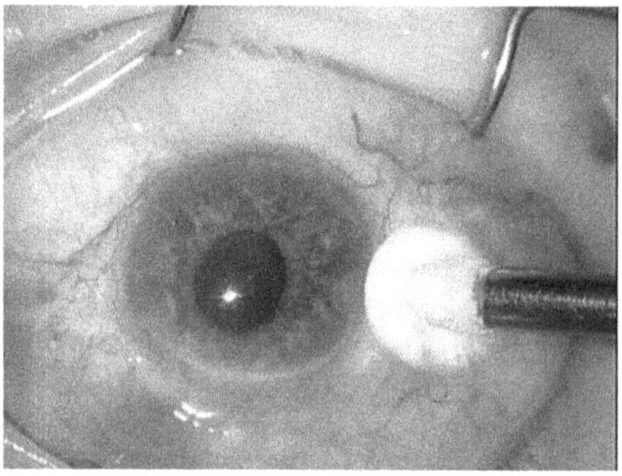

Fig. 13.2 A cryopexy of the ciliary body. The cryo probe is placed correctly if ¼ of the cryo effect affects the cornea and ¾ the limbus

In the most cases, the IOP reduces significantly within 4 weeks: If the IOP decreased below 35 mmHg we perform only a retinal cryopexy and no cryopexy of the ciliary body. If the IOP is over 35 mmHg we place 2–4 cryopexy spots in the inferior half of the ciliary body (Fig. 13.2). Remark: Be cautious with cryopexy of ciliary body as it may result in hypotony.

13.2 The Surgery

Instruments

1. **Chandelier light fibre.**
2. **BIOM with 120D lens.**
3. **Cryopexy handpiece.**

Individual steps

1. **Limbal peritomy.**
2. **Insertion of chandelier light fibre.**
3. **Retinal cryopexy under BIOM view.**

4. Cryopexy of ciliary body under microscope view.
5. Reposition of conjunctiva.

The surgery step by step:

1. Limbal peritomy.
2. Insertion of chandelier light fibre.

Begin with a 360° limbal peritomy. Then insert a chandelier light at the inferotemporal or nasal position (Fig. 13.3).

3. Retinal cryopexy under BIOM view

Flick in the BIOM and perform a circular cryopexy (Fig. 13.4). We freeze first the retina on the height of the equator and then continue to freeze the retina between equator and the temporal arcades. The freezing time depends on the cryo device you are using. It is approximately 5–10 seconds. Wait until you see a white bleaching of the retina.

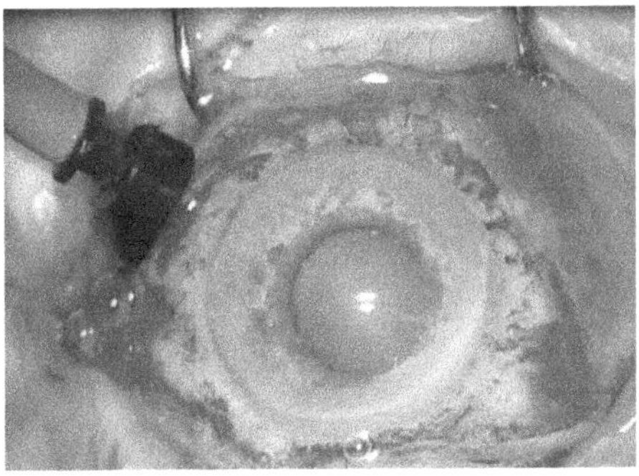

Fig. 13.3 A cryopexy of the retina. Perform a 360° limbal peritomy and insert a chandelier light. The limbal peritomy prevents damage of conjunctival goblet cells

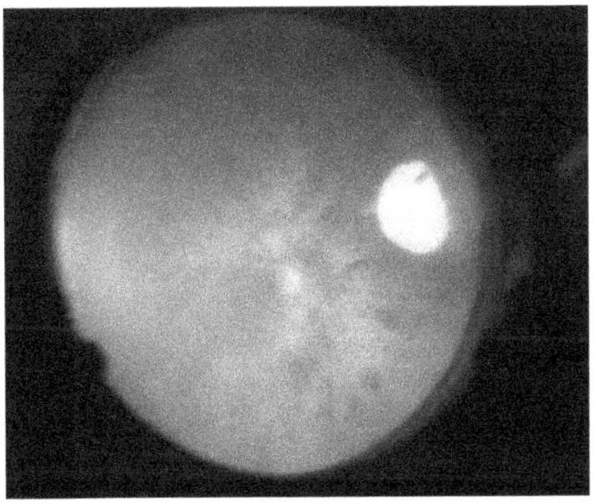

Fig. 13.4 Flick in the BIOM to visualize the retina. The view to fundus is much better with the microscope than with binocular indirect ophthalmoscopy. Freeze the retina with the cryopexy handpiece until you observe a good bleaching, approximately 10 s

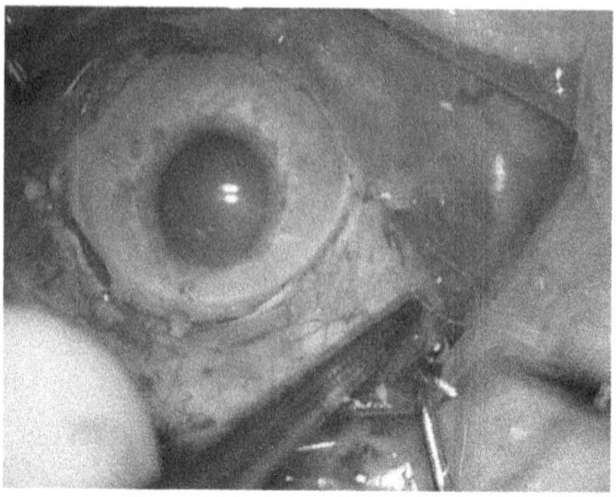

Fig. 13.5 Close the conjunctiva with Vicryl 8-0

4. Cryopexy of ciliary body under microscope view
Proceed with cryopexy of the ciliary body. We freeze the inferior half of the ciliary body and spare the superior half in order to avoid hypotony. We freeze 30 seconds. This depends again on the cryopexy device. Depending on the tip size of the cryopexy handpiece you can place 2–3 freezings per quadrant (Fig. 13.2). The cryopexy areas should be adjacent to each other.

5. Reposition of conjunctiva
Remove the chandelier light fibre. Close the sclerotomy with a Vicryl-8-0 suture. Inject 0.1 ml bevacizumab intravitreal. Then close the conjunctiva at 3 and 9 o'clock with a Vicryl-8–0 suture (Fig. 13.5).

Part VII

Surgical Failures and Postoperative Complications

All videos of this book are found on the Youtube channel from Ulrich Spandau and playing list "Proliferative diabetic retinopathy" (link: https://youtube.com/playlist?list=PL0dKYclPD7yM9qRjBoF1HMwtxFfbf2T6A).

Section 14.1: "Easy" PDR with completely attached posterior hyaloid

Section 14.2: Retinal detachment after cryopexy

Section 14.3: Retinal defects after difficult PDR

Section 14.4: Hypotony after several vitreoretinal surgeries secondary to PDR

Section 14.5: Displacement of the macula after resorption of SUBRETINAL FLUID

Chapter 15: Postsurgical complications

Surgical Failures 14

In this part, we present surgical failures. You can learn a lot from your surgical failures. Learn from your first mistake and avoid the same mistake a second time.

14.1 "Easy" PDR with Completely Attached Posterior Hyaloid

This complication is very tricky because you do not expect it. The typical patient is a 60–70 y/o patient with type 2 diabetes. A moderate non-proliferative diabetic retinopathy is present. The indication for surgery may be an epiretinal membrane or a vitreous hemorrhage. You start surgery and realize that no PVD is present. When you induce a posterior vitreous detachment, it gets very difficult because the posterior hyaloid is firmly attached. A PVD up to the equator is difficult. These eyes may experience severe postoperative complications in form of vitreous hemorrhage and PVR detachment.

The following case will explain and illustrate my experience:

A 58 y/o female patient with type 2 diabetes and 3× vitreous hemorrhage within 8 months and treated with scatter laser (PRP). One month before vitrectomy Eylea is injected. A lens-sparing vitrectomy is performed. Peroperative the posterior vitreous is completely attached (Fig. 14.1). A careful PVD is induced. The PVD can only be induced up to the equator due to strong adherence. A fill-in PRP is done. Six weeks later a moderate vitreous hemorrhage is observed and the peripheral retina is attached. A combined lavage vitrectomy is scheduled. Six weeks later, one day before the scheduled vitrectomy, a severe PVR retinal detachment is detected (Fig. 14.2). The patient reports that her diabetes deteriorated and that a kidney and pancreas transplant is planned. A combined phaco/vitrectomy is performed. The anterior vitreous is very bloody. Several PVR membranes are removed and the retina is reattached under silicone oil. In the following 3 months, PVR reoccurs and two more vitrectomies have to be performed.

U. Spandau and Z. Tomic, *Small-Gauge Vitrectomy for Diabetic Retinopathy*,
https://doi.org/10.1007/978-3-031-26204-3_14

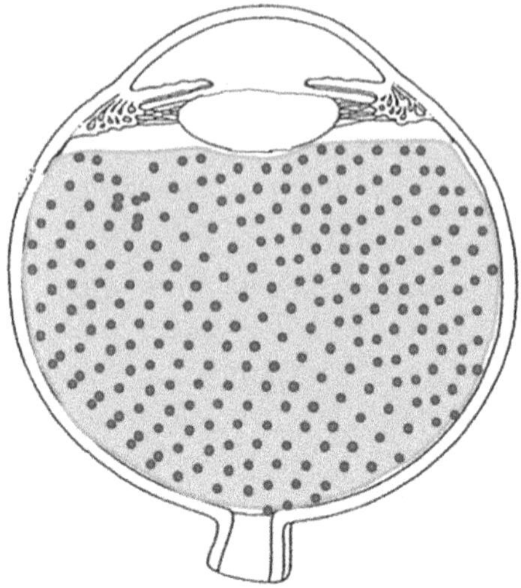

Fig. 14.1 Surgical situation prior first surgery. The eye has a natural lens, a vitreous hemorrhage is present and the posterior vitreous is attached

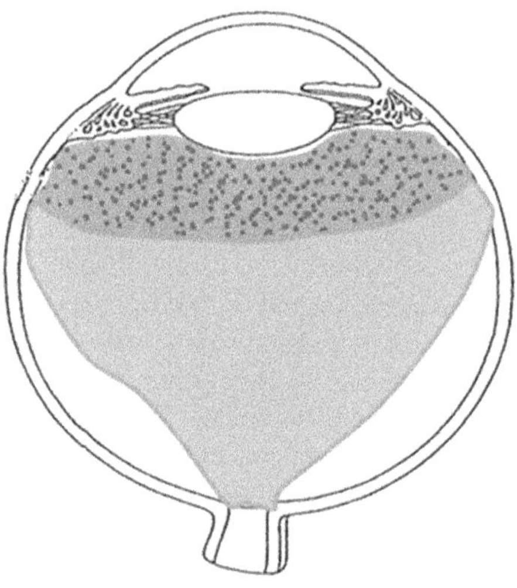

Fig. 14.2 Surgical situation prior second surgery. The eye has a natural lens, an anterior vitreous hemorrhage is present and a total tractive retinal detachment is present

The same complication happened to me when I operated a 72 y/o female patient for epiretinal membrane (Fig. 14.3). She had a simplex retinopathy and no scatter laser. The posterior vitreous was completely attached (Fig. 14.4). A PVD was very difficult because the posterior hyaloid was very adherent to the retina from posterior to anterior. I managed to induce a PVD up to the equator and then removed the epiretinal membrane. In the postoperative course, she developed a PVR detachment.

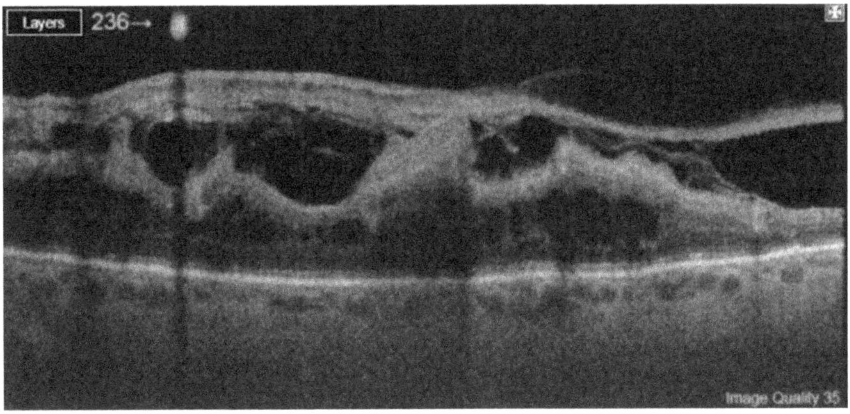

Fig. 14.3 An old patient with diabetic retinopathy. OCT, showing several adhesions between posterior hyaloid and retina

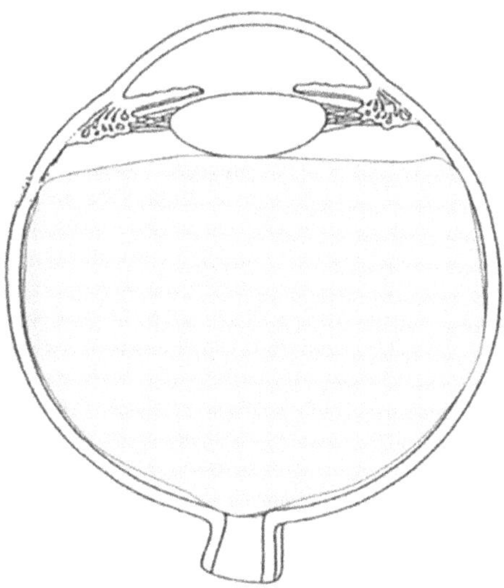

Fig. 14.4 This 72 y/o patient was planned for epiretinal membrane removal. A mild diabetic retinopathy was present. But the posterior hyaloid was firmly attached

With a hindsight of 20/20 would you have done things differently?
Yes, I would not perform a lens-sparing vitrectomy. I would start with phaco and anti-VEGF and perform 4 weeks later a vitrectomy in order to remove the complete anterior vitreous during the first surgery.

14.2 Retinal Detachment After Cryopexy

In my surgical career, I performed two times a retinal cryopexy in patients with advanced PDR. Both times a retinal detachment occurred. With a hindsight of

20/20 I am today very hesitant with cryopexy in patients with PDR. Cryopexy has a high PVR risk. In contrast, I have never experienced a PVR detachment after laser photocoagulation.

The following case report illustrates my experience:

A very sick 23-year-old female patient, type I diabetic with multiple comorbidities, heart failure, kidney failure and drug addiction was hospitalized in 09/2013 due to ketoacidosis. During the hospital visit she was examined by the ophthalmological department due to bilateral severe visual impairment. Visual acuity was hand movement and a PDR with high-risk characteristic, advanced retinal ischemia and preretinal fibrosis was diagnosed. An angiography revealed on the LE extensive retinal ischemia involving the macula (Fig. 14.5). The eye was not scatter laser treated. I decided to treat the eye with a retinal cryopexy. First an Avastin injection was given. One month later a retinal cryopexy was performed. Two weeks later a total retinal detachment was observed (Fig. 14.6). A vitrectomy was performed and the retina was reattached with silicone oil (Figs. 14.7 and 14.8).

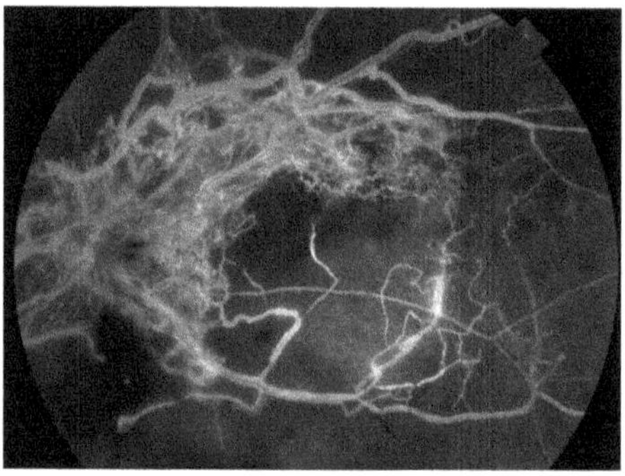

Fig. 14.5 Left eye. Angiography reveals extreme ischemia. Visual function is 0.05

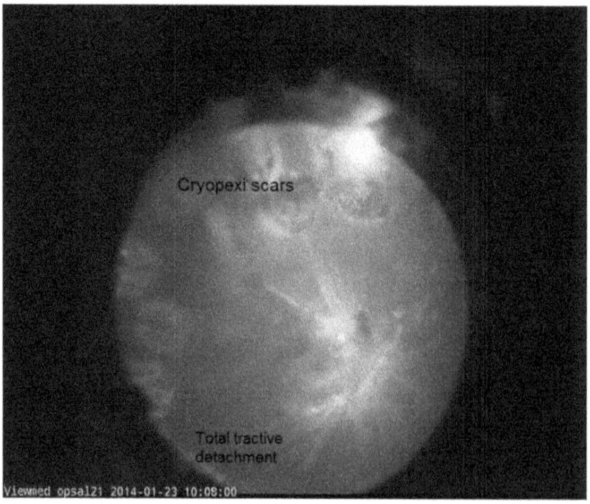

Fig. 14.6 A total retinal detachment after cryopexy treatment

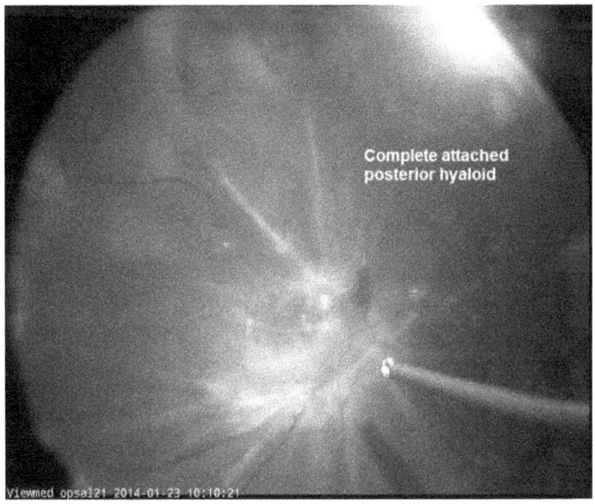

Fig. 14.7 The posterior hyaloid is attached. It has to be removed completely

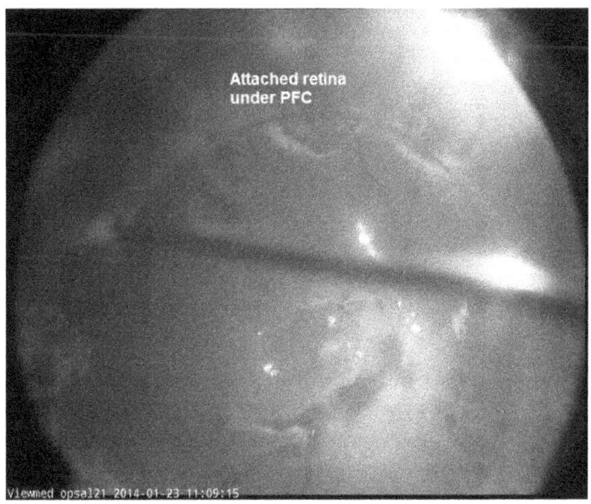

Fig. 14.8 The posterior hyaloid is removed in the centre and in the periphery. PFCL is injected to attach the detached retina. The retina remains attached under 5000 cSt silicone oil

14.3 Retinal Defects After Complicated Vitrectomy

Huge retinal defects during diabetic vitrectomy are a serious complication. I observed this serious complication in two VR clinics. Both VR clinics do not treat their patients with anti-VEGF prior surgery.

The following cases illustrate my observation:

Case 1:
A 56 y/o male patient presented with a PDR with tractive retinal detachment in the right eye. The eye was never treated with scatter laser or anti-VEGF. No pre-treatment before vitrectomy was performed (Fig. 14.9). The vitrectomy included

a peeling, laser and silicone oil tamponade. During membrane removal huge retinal defects occurred. The result can be seen in Fig. 14.10. The silicone oil is left permanently in the eye.

Case 2:
A 43 y/o male patient presented with a tractive retinal detachment in the right eye. The eye was never treated with scatter laser or with anti-VEGF. No pretreatment before vitrectomy was performed. During peeling a huge retinal defect in the nasal pole occurred. A permanent silicone oil tamponade was applied (Fig. 14.11).

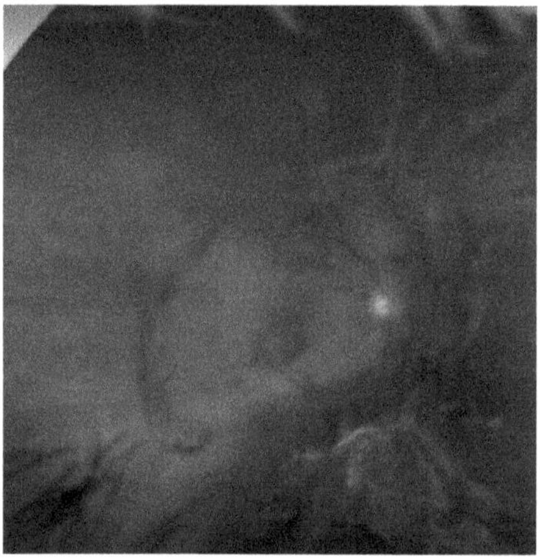

Fig. 14.9 First case. Before surgery. A PDR with nasal and inferior TRD

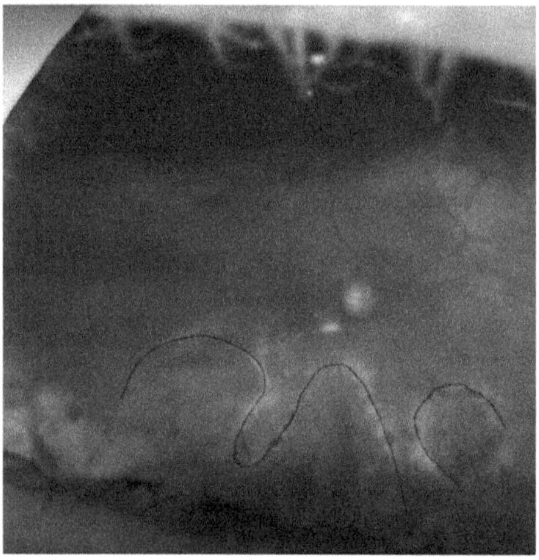

Fig. 14.10 First case. After surgery: Postoperative picture with silicone-filled eye. Note the huge retinal defects in the inferior pole after traumatic peeling

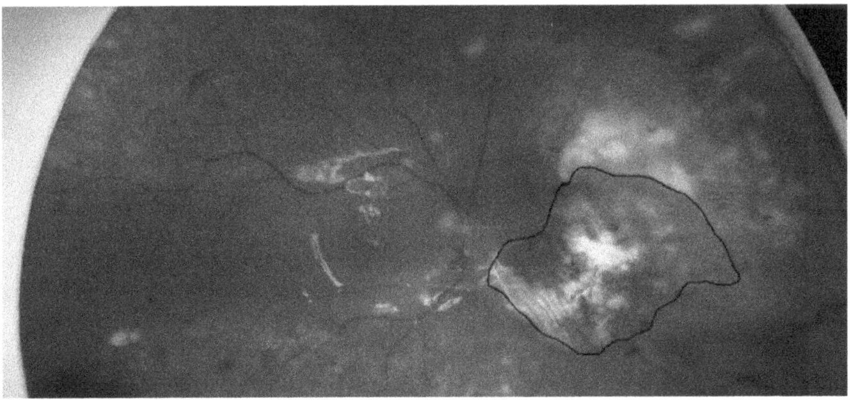

Fig. 14.11 Second case. Postoperative picture with permanent silicone-filled eye. Note the huge retinal defect in the nasal pole after traumatic peeling

Case 3:
No general clinical data available. A patient with a severe PDR was operated with vitrectomy and ILM peeling. No anti-VEGF treatment was given before or during surgery. One month later the retina was completely detached (Fig. 14.12). An advanced PVR was present.

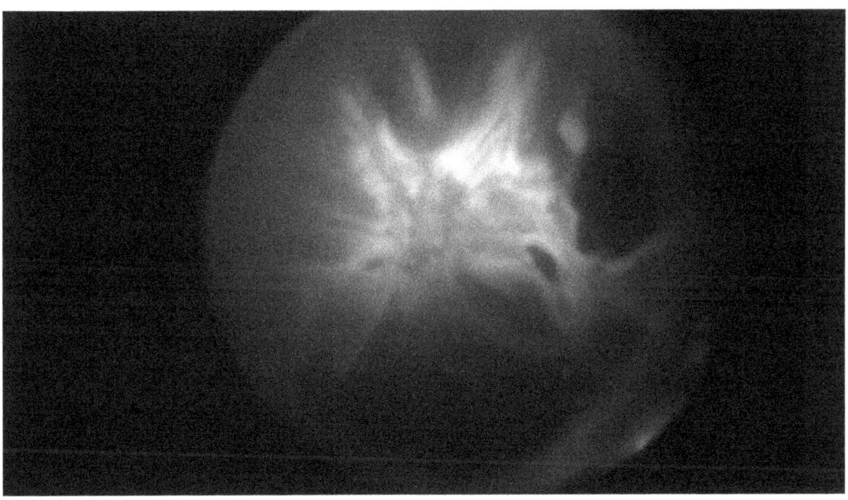

Fig. 14.12 Third case: 1-month after vitrectomy for diabetic retinopathy. Note the huge retinal defect. No anti-VEGF treatment was given before or during surgery

Conclusion: Quieten an angry PDR before vitrectomy. Otherwise, you will create large retinal defects and secondly you will have many patients with permanent silicone oil tamponade (Figs. 14.10 and 14.11).

14.4 Hypotony After Several Vitreoretinal Surgeries Secondary to PDR

Hypotony after several vitreoretinal surgeries is a dreaded complication and considered as failure. Please read the following case and avoid the mistakes made here.

A 41-year-old male patient with type I diabetes. He presented to our clinic due to VA reduction to 0.01 on the right eye. The left eye had a visual acuity of 0.7. The right eye had a severe proliferative diabetic retinopathy. The patient had a bad compliance, both eyes never treated with anti-VEGF or scatter laser. The surgical video of the *right* eye is available under this link: https://youtu.be/TGCdPToL1bk.

Both eyes were first treated with bilateral Avastin injections. In the **first surgery,** the right eye was treated with combined phaco/vitrectomy + peeling + laser + silicone oil + Avastin (Figs. 14.13, 14.14, 14.15 and 14.16). During the postoperative follow-up, the visual acuity improved to 0,4. Due to a bad regulation of his diabetes the eye became again proliferative and membranes reoccurred. Therefore, two surgeries were performed with silicone oil extraction + peeling + laser + silicone oil (**second and third surgeries**). The diabetic retinopathy quietened but the IOP increased to 40 mmHg. The silicone oil was consequently removed (**fourth surgery**) but the IOP did not decrease and a central detachment occurred. The eye was therefore operated with cryopexy of the ciliary body + peeling and injection of silicone oil (**fifth surgery**). In the postoperative follow-up, the eye developed a hypotony and a recurrence of subretinal membranes. In the **final** surgery, the membranes were removed (**sixth surgery**). Since then the eye is stable with a VA = HM, the diabetic retinopathy has not reoccurred but the silicone oil was not removed due to a low pressure of 6 mmHg (Fig. 14.17). The **table** in Fig. 14.18 shows the development of IOP during a 4-year treatment period.

With a hindsight of 20/20 would you have done things differently?
I operated this patient in the beginning of my surgical career (US). Today, I would treat the patient differently. I would perform a stepwise surgery. First phaco and Avastin and then a PRP in the out-patient department or a LIO in general anaesthesia. I would try to delay the vitrectomy for a few months after laser treatment, but I would definitely perform a vitrectomy. I doubt that the secondary glaucoma would have occurred with my new treatment planning. Nowadays, I treat a secondary glaucoma with an Ahmed valve and not with cryopexy of the ciliary body.

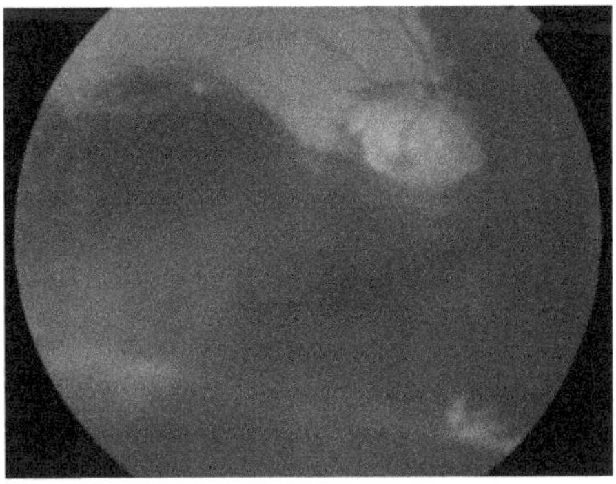

Fig. 14.13 Right eye of a type I diabetic with poor compliance and no pretreatment. Advanced PDR and subhyaloidal hemorrhage

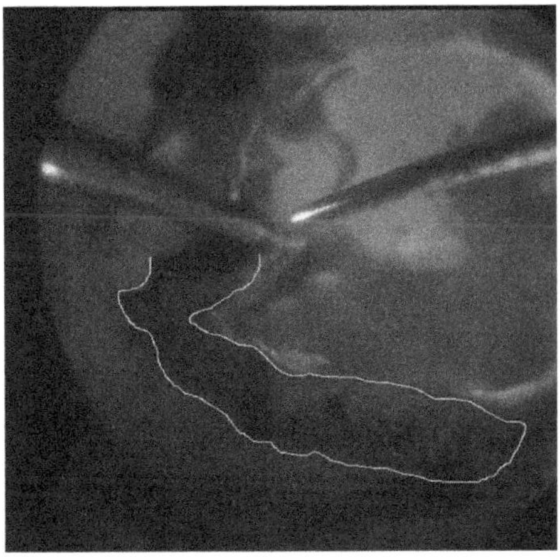

Fig. 14.14 RE: Intraoperative image of a posterior hyaloid rhexis

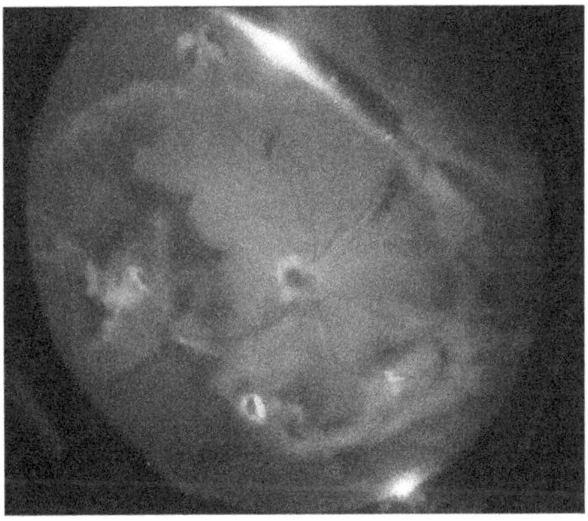

Fig. 14.15 RE: Intraoperative image after removal of membranes

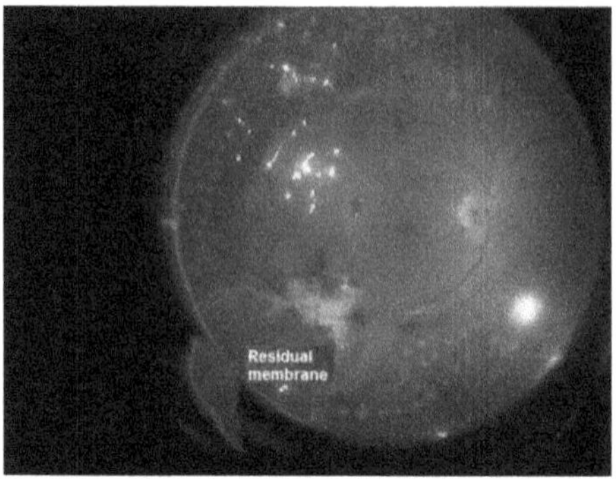

Fig. 14.16 RE: Intraoperative image after PRP and injection of 1000 cSt silicone oil

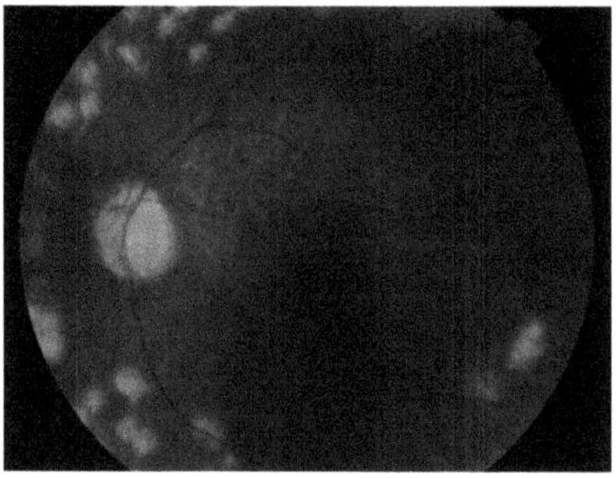

Fig. 14.17 RE: Final 2-year follow-up. Vitreous cavity is filled with silicone oil due to hypotony. The VA is reduced due to an optic atrophy. VA = HM, IOP = 7 mmHg

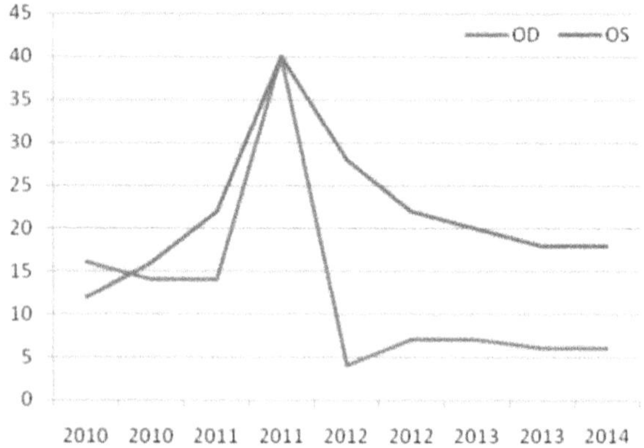

Fig. 14.18 IOP of right eye (OD) and left eye (OS). The first surgery was 2010

14.5 Displacement of the Macula After Resorption of Subretinal Fluid

The issue of displacement of the macula after resorption of subretinal fluid where there was a high TRD is an interesting one. In our opinion, we don't think there is much one can do to prevent it. Maybe the acute flattening during air-fluid exchange makes the displacement worse, but, even in cases where there are no breaks and where no tamponade at all is used, and where the subretinal fluid then slowly resorbs over time, sometimes there is still displacement. Maybe the chronic high traction causes an element of stretching of the retina with loss of elasticity, which causes it to just always want to sag down. We are not convinced that the tamponading agent makes a difference, and we think that the risk of other complications with silicone oil tamponade (and the burden of an additional surgery to remove the SO) outweigh the burden of this complication.

Case report: 30 y/o female patient with type 1 diabetes and poor compliance. A ring-formed TRD is present (Fig. 14.19). After vitrectomy, an inferior displacement of the superior arcade was observed (Fig. 14.20).

Abstract
A difficult surgery such as diabetic retinopathy has often postsurgical complications. The following chapter describes the management of postsurgical complications after vitrectomy.

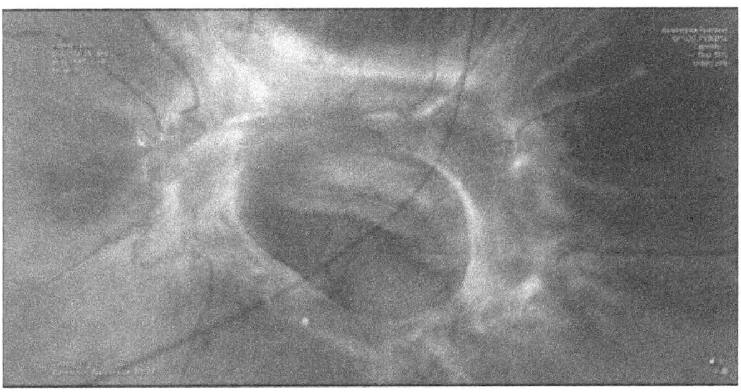

Fig. 14.19 Preoperative fundus. The tractions did not aggravate after anti-VEGF injection

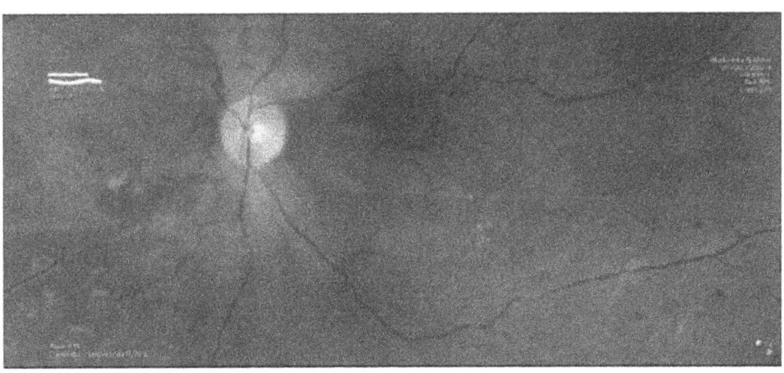

Fig. 14.20 Postoperative fundus 3 months after vitrectomy. Note that the superior arcade is inferiorly dislocated and the macula has a fold

14.6 Surgery of an Eye with Iris Rubeosis

Case report: An 88 y/o male patient presents with iris rubeosis and 2 mm hyphema. IOP is 45 mmHg and vision is light perception. The fundus shows an ischemic retinopathy secondary to CRVO with attached retina and pale optic disc. The plan was removal of blood from anterior chamber and retinal cryopexy.

During surgery there was more blood than expected in the anterior chamber. The iris rubeosis bled continuously during surgery. A chandelier light was inserted and a retinal cryopexy under BIOM view was performed.

Two days postoperative, the patient returned with an IOP of 56 mmHg and 90% hyphema. The patient is treated with intravenous and oral IOP lowering medication, the IOP reduced to 42 mmHg. After 6 weeks postoperative, the IOP reduced to 22 mmHg.

With hindsight of 20/20 would you have done things differently?
Do not operate on an eye with iris rubeosis. Inject first intravitreal anti-VEGF, wait 4 weeks and perform then a retinal cryopexy. With this treatment planning I never again had this complication.

Postoperative Complications and Management

15

Intraoperative retinal hemorrhage.
If the retina bleeds very much and you are not able to stop the bleeding then use following approach: Abandon the removal of fibrovascular membranes, do a fill-in PRP, continue with a fluid-air exchange and inject anti-VEGF. Schedule the next surgery in 1–3 months. In case of excessive peroperative bleeding we recommend the same procedure but a silicone oil tamponade.

Early and late postoperative vitreous hemorrhage:
The cause for postoperative hemorrhage is the washout of blood cells from the residual vitreous gel and bleeding from neovascular retinal vessels. In case of a lens-sparing vitrectomy, the washout is bigger because the anterior vitreous is not removed. You can reduce the washout of blood cells if you perform a phacoemulsification, remove all anterior vitreous and cauterize meticulously all bleeding sources with endodiathermy.

An *early* vitreous hemorrhage is common if you do not treat diabetic patients preoperatively and peroperatively with anti-VEGF. Since we use anti-VEGF as a standard regime for surgery we could reduce the rate of early postoperative hemorrhage to almost zero. A *late* vitreal hemorrhage, however, may occur many months after surgery. In this case, we do not perform a lavage vitrectomy but schedule a course of three anti-VEGF injections. A lavage is a vitrectomy with aspiration of intraocular blood and an air tamponade.

Postoperative bleed in a silicone-filled eye.
A big postoperative bleed on the posterior pole may occur. The silicone oil prevents that the blood disperses into the posterior segment and presses it against the posterior pole. The epiretinal blood will disappear within 4 weeks. It will first liquIfy and then sink to the inferior part of the vitreous cavity and finally resorb (this can take an additional 4–8 weeks). We recommend to remove the silicone

U. Spandau and Z. Tomic, *Small-Gauge Vitrectomy for Diabetic Retinopathy*,
https://doi.org/10.1007/978-3-031-26204-3_15

oil with residual blood after 3 months. **Remark**: If you experience a significant bleeding during surgery then choose a silicone oil tamponade and not gas.

IOP rise:
An IOP rise can have many reasons. It may be caused by the tamponade or the combination of a bleeding and tamponade; a strong postoperative bleed in a silicone-oil-filled eye results in an increased IOP. A silicone oil tamponade requires a tight IOP control such as every second week. A neovascularization of the iris (NVI) results in a neovascular glaucoma. In the latter case, we inject anti-VEGF immediately in order to reduce the NVI. In a second step, the neovascular stimulus must be suppressed with laser or cryopexy. Please see the chapter in this book "Neovascular glaucoma". Young phakic patients with silicone oil tamponade have an increased risk for high IOP. If a glaucoma surgery is necessary, we implant an Ahmed valve. Remove the silicone oil after maximal 3 months.

Gas tamponade:
The disadvantage of a gas tamponade is the bad view to fundus. This problem aggravates in case of a peroperative hemorrhage. If you use a long-lasting gas you will have no view to the fundus for 2 months. We recommend Sf_6 and C_2F_6 for diabetic eyes. Other clinics prefer C_3F_8. Generally, we recommend a gas tamponade for diabetic patients. But in case of extensive bleeding under the surgery, we recommend a silicone oil tamponade.

New membranes:
Membranes may recur after vitrectomy. Reasons are an incomplete removal of membranes in the initial vitrectomy or a reactivation of the diabetic retinopathy with a growth of new membranes. If the membranes cause tractions then they have to be removed. Perform an anti-VEGF injection to quieten the retina and schedule a second vitrectomy.

Reoperate the eye. Check, if the posterior hyaloid is completely removed. Remove the membranes and perform a fill-in PRP.

Recurrent neovascularization of iris (NVI):
Neovascularization of iris is caused by a persistent neovascular stimulus. The stimulus has to be suppressed with anti-VEGF and laser treatment.

If a neovascularization of the iris is present and the retina is treated with a scatter laser then the most common reason is an incomplete PRP. In the most cases, there is no scatter laser from the equator to the ora serrata because a laser treatment at the slit lamp goes only to the equator. Many dense PRPs at the slit lamp are not so dense under BIOM view. Perform a vitrectomy and laser treat the retina between equator and ora serrata.

If the retina is treated with a PRP up to the ora serrata and nonetheless you observe a recurrent or persistent iris rubeosis, then the PRP is not dense enough. If an eye has NVI, then it has residual ischemic retina and is not sufficiently laser treated. Perform a vitrectomy with fill-in PRP from the temporal arcade up to the ora serrata and inject Avastin. Wait 3 months for the surgical effect. An alternative is a LIO treatment in general anaesthesia.

In advanced cases of neovascular glaucoma without useful function cryopexy can be used.

Anti-VEGF injection in an eye with high IOP.

An injection of 0.05 anti-VEGF solution into an eye with high IOP is no problem. We performed injection in eyes with IOP of 54 mmHg without any problem. We do not perform an AC tap. *Remark*: Be careful with an injection in a small eye (microphthalmia). To avoid an excessive IOP increase give the patient 500 mg acetazolomide 2 hours before injection.

Part VIII
Case Reports

All videos of this book are found on the Youtube channel from Ulrich Spandau and playing list "Proliferative diabetic retinopathy" (link: https://youtube.com/playlist?list=PL0dKYclPD7yM9qRjBoF1HMwtxFfbf2T6A).

Chapter 16: Case reports

Swedish patients:

First case report: No video available

Second case report: https://youtu.be/2smIKSoEgDw

Third case report: https://youtu.be/jMWeLFefgbk

Fourth case report: https://youtu.be/cSA7ZAuO6aM

Fifth case report: https://youtu.be/wNueV3Z1ZIU

Serbian patients:

Sixth case report: https://youtu.be/FhPp4FqriI0 and https://youtu.be/BOe8bgFSlao

Seventh case report: https://youtu.be/LNEvbtqQCRo

Eighth case report: https://youtu.be/FFr1KKwbsBE

Ninth case report: https://youtu.be/UA5mhE1l7O4

Tenth case report: https://youtu.be/9yg4e6P7nkU

Case Reports

16

The patient collective you see and treat as an ophthalmologist is very much dependent of the national health system. Patients with chronic diseases such as glaucoma and diabetes are most dependent on good and regular ward. The quality of the diabetic screening is reflected by the severity of diabetic retinopathy you encounter in your operating room. This can be very well observed in the following case reports from Sweden with a rigid centralized diabetic screening and Serbia with a practically none existing diabetic screening.

The following case reports are from Sweden (Case 1–Case 5) and from former Yugoslavia (Serbia) (Case 6–Case 10).

16.1 Swedish Patients

The **Swedish** healthcare system is dominated by state-owned hospitals and polyclinic centres. There are only a few private ophthalmologists. The screening and treatment of diabetic patients is almost completely in the hand of the hospitals. Only the eye department of the University of Uppsala is responsible for the screening and treatment of all patients in her province. The province of Uppsala has 350.000 inhabitants and the department of ophthalmology screens 3500 diabetic patients per year. The vast majority of patients receive a timely and complete treatment; a minority of patients—especially diabetics with a low compliance—fall through the screening net and receive no treatment whatsoever until they meet you for the first time. This is especially the case for young type I diabetics with low compliance; Scandinavia is known to have a high prevalence of type I diabetics.

First case report: Bilateral PDR treated with LIO and vitrectomy
The following case shows the strengths of our stepwise treatment planning:

A 30 y/o male patient with type 1 diabetes. This case shows the positive effect of our treatment planning with intravitreal Lucentis and laser photocoagulation in two eyes with PDR, retinal proliferations and vitreous hemorrhage (Figs. 16.1, 16.2, 16.3,

U. Spandau and Z. Tomic, *Small-Gauge Vitrectomy for Diabetic Retinopathy*,
https://doi.org/10.1007/978-3-031-26204-3_16

16.4, 16.5 and 16.6, **case 1**). The effect is only positive and no complications occur. I hope this case can reduce your fear for using anti-VEGF in patients with PDR.

I have *no surgical video* available on this case.

Second case report: Severe TRD

A 45 y/o male patient with insulin-dependent diabetes present with an extensive macula threatening TRD. The eye was first treated with phaco and Avastin and 1 month later with vitrectomy (Figs. 16.7, 16.8, 16.9 and 16.10, **case 2**).

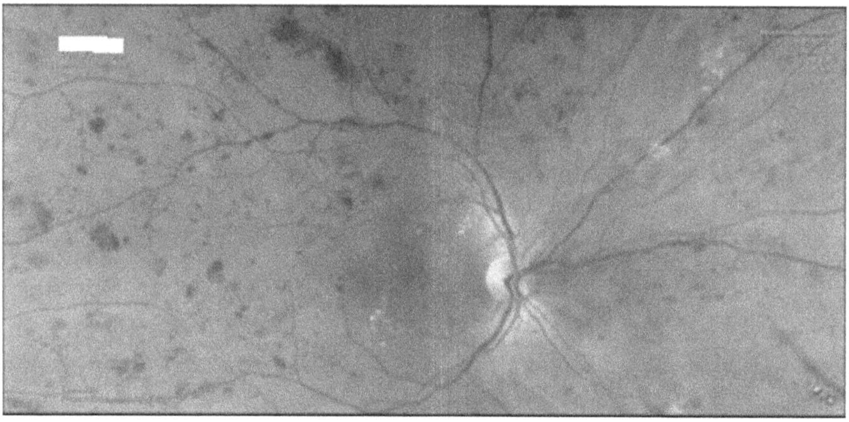

Fig. 16.1 **Case 1**: Right eye. An Optos photograph of the preoperative fundus. Note the retinal proliferations

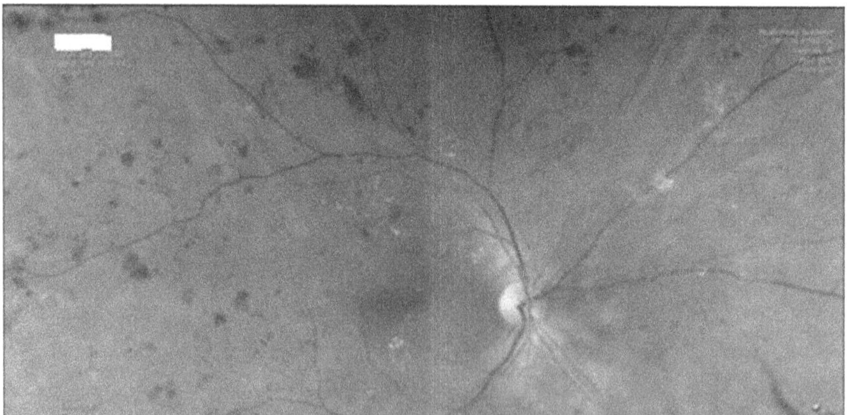

Fig. 16.2 **Case 1**: Right eye. An Optos photograph one month after Lucentis injection. The retinal proliferations are gone. No tractions visible. A LIO was scheduled

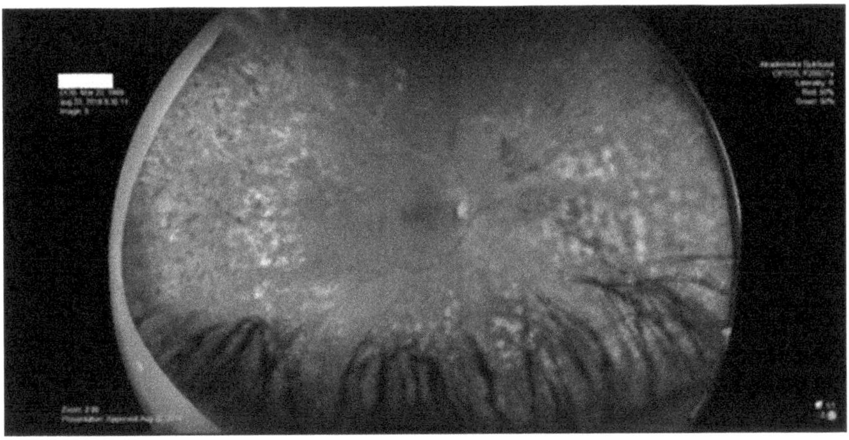

Fig. 16.3 **Case 1**: Right eye. An Optos photograph of the retina 2 months after LIO

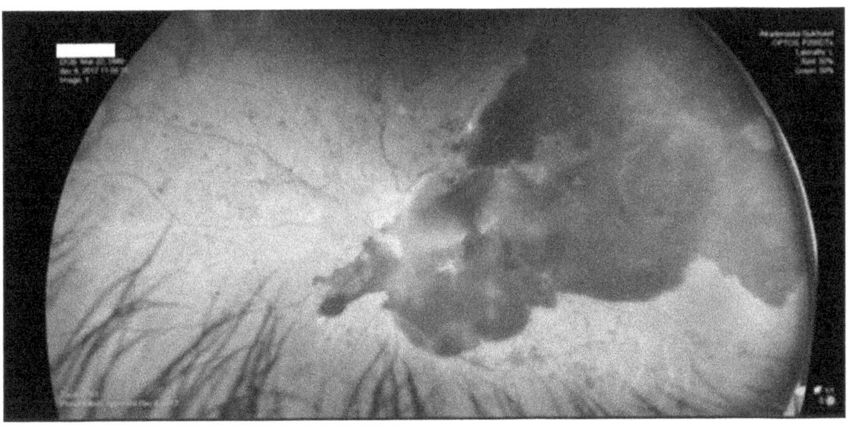

Fig. 16.4 **Case 1**: Left eye: An Optos photograph of the preoperative fundus. Note the sub-hyaloidal hemorrhage

The surgical video of this case is available under this link: https://youtu.be/2smIKSoEgDw.

With a hindsight of 20/20 would you have done things differently?

This macula threatening TRD contracted partially after anti-VEGF injection (crunch effect). The macula was not affected. Today, I would operate the eye earlier or do a weekly follow-up.

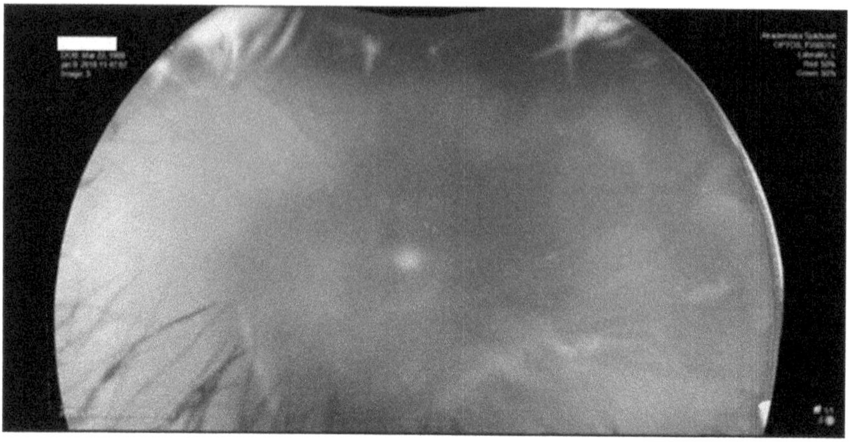

Fig. 16.5 **Case 1**: Left eye: 1 month after Lucentis injection. The hemorrhage has entered the vitreous gel. No tractions are visible. A vitrectomy was scheduled

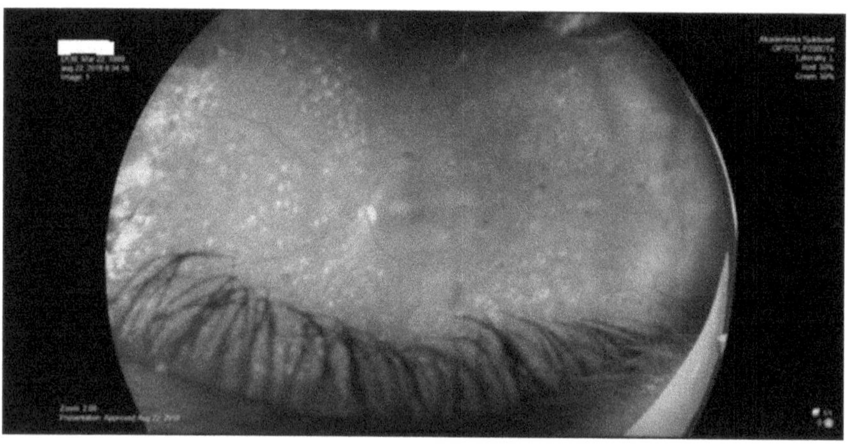

Fig. 16.6 **Case 1**: Left eye: 2 months after vitrectomy

Third case report: Severe PDR and TRD

A 34y/o male war refugee with insulin-dependent diabetes experienced a severe VA loss in his right eye (hand movement). A severe PDR with TRD was diagnosed. Both eyes were first treated with LIO and Avastin. Three weeks later surgery was scheduled (Fig. 16.11, **case 3**). A 27G lens-sparing vitrectomy was performed. Surgery was finalized with a 15% C2F6 gas tamponade and Avastin injection. The postoperative VA after 3 months was 0.4 (Fig. 16.11, **case 3**).

The surgical video of this case is available under this link: https://youtu.be/jMWeLFefgbk.

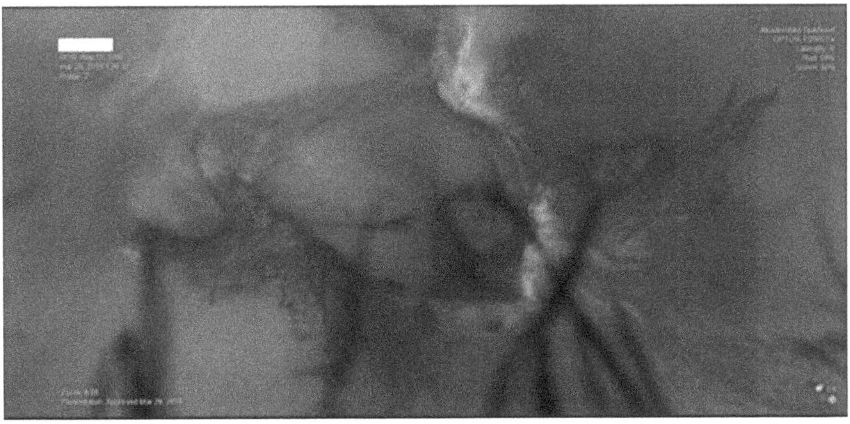

Fig. 16.7 **Case 2:** An Optos photograph of the preoperative fundus. Never laser treated. Note the extensive proliferations. Would you not pretreat this eye? Or rather deal with intraoperative bleeding?

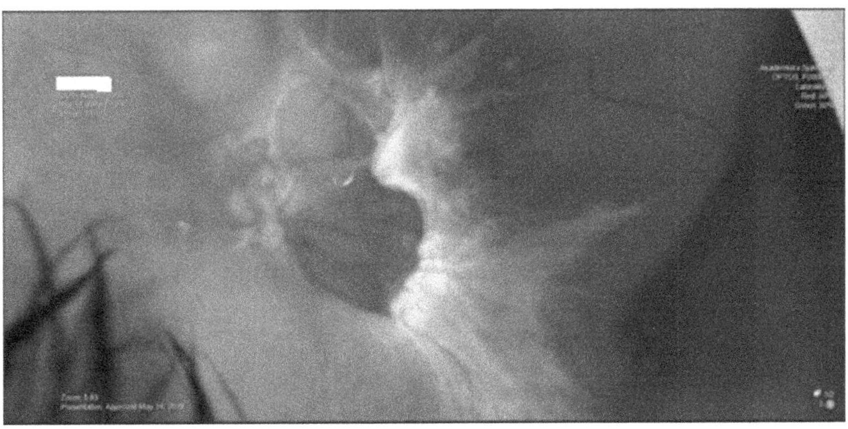

Fig. 16.8 **Case 2:** An Optos photograph one month after phaco and Avastin. Note the marked reduction of proliferations. Note also the detached retina temporal to the membranes

With a hindsight of 20/20 would you have done things differently?

No. The surgical video shows very well that a preoperative treatment reduces vitrectomy times, reduces number of endodiathermy effects, minimizes retinal tears and speeds up postoperative visual recovery.

Fourth case report: Severe TRD
A 42 y/o male patient with insulin-dependent diabetes and two amputated legs. He was never laser treated in his eyes. Visual acuity was RE = 0.6 and LE = 0.1 (Fig. 16.12, **case 4**). Both eyes received a Lucentis injection and were treated with

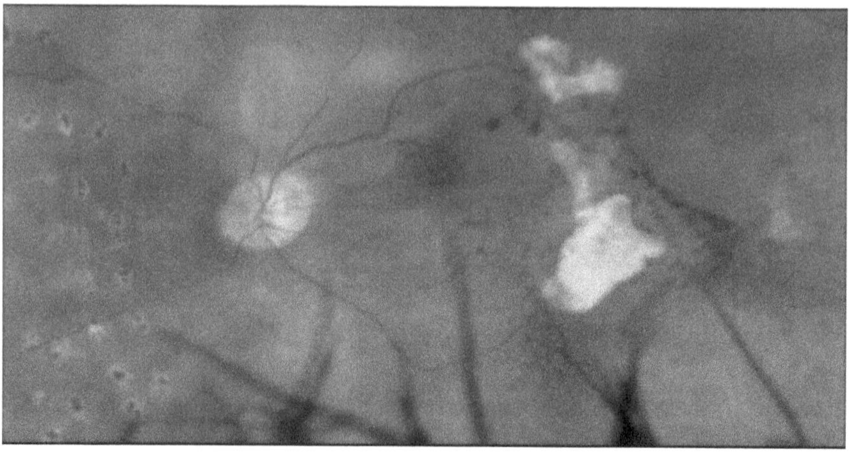

Fig. 16.9 **Case 2:** Two months after vitrectomy. The white remnants are residual membranes. It was unclear whether this was retinal tissue or not. They were not removed, please note that they do not create any traction longer because there are no tissue bridges between them

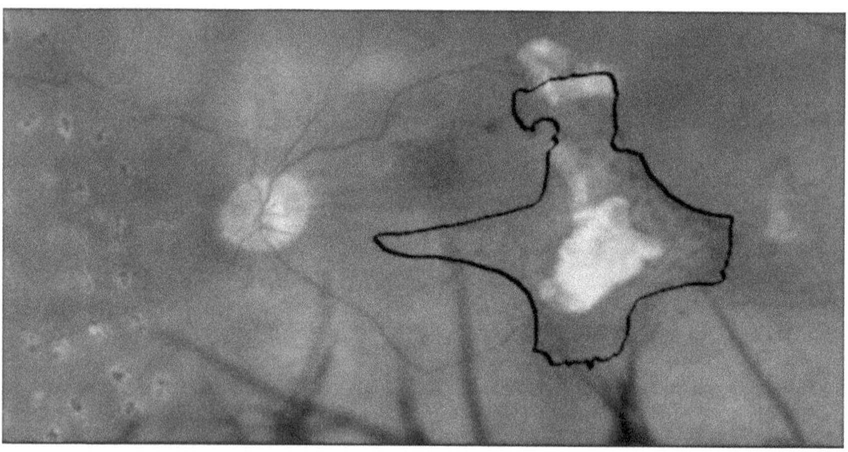

Fig. 16.10 **Case 2:** The black marked area was detached preoperatively. Note that the macula remained attached

laser indirect ophthalmoscopy (LIO). Two weeks later the patient presented with a visual acuity decrease in his left eye. The macula had detached (Figs. 16.13 and 16.14, **case 4**). An immediate vitrectomy was scheduled. Two weeks postoperative the VA was 0.05 (Fig. 16.15, **case 4**).

The surgical video of this case is available under this link: https://youtu.be/cSA7ZAuO6aM.

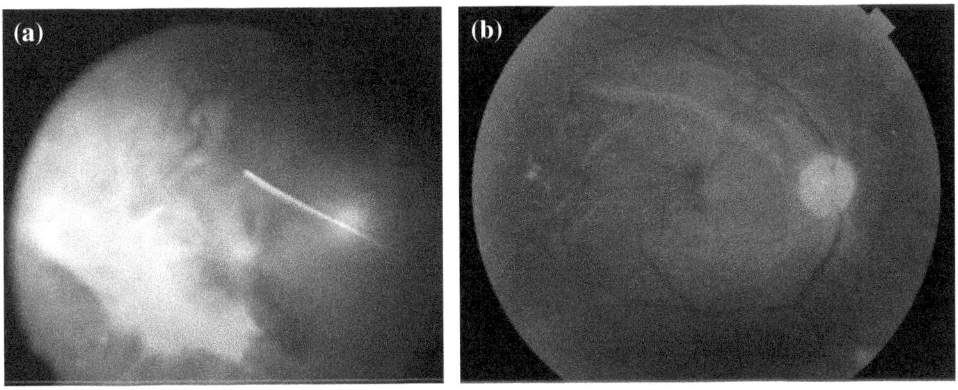

Fig. 16.11 **Case 3:** (a): A peroperative photograph of the fundus. (b): A postperative photograph

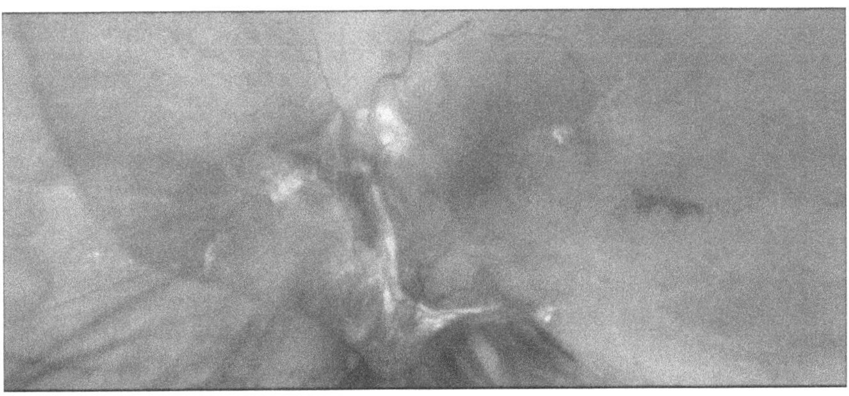

Fig. 16.12 **Case 4:** Preoperative fundus

With a hindsight of 20/20 would you have done things differently?

This case is the only case in my surgical career in which the macula detached after an anti-VEGF injection. It cannot however be excluded that the laser photocoagulation was responsible or even the natural course had yielded the same result. I would not alter my treatment planning. Why? I prefer to have a safe surgery and avoid a surgical failure.

Fifth case report: Extensive subhyaloidal hemorrhage
A 48-year-old male patient, he is severe ill, has type 2 diabetes, both legs amputated, renal failure and heavy smoker. He was admitted to our clinic due to severe PDR in both eyes. Please note that both eyes are treated on every occasion.

2014-01-02: Presurgical examination

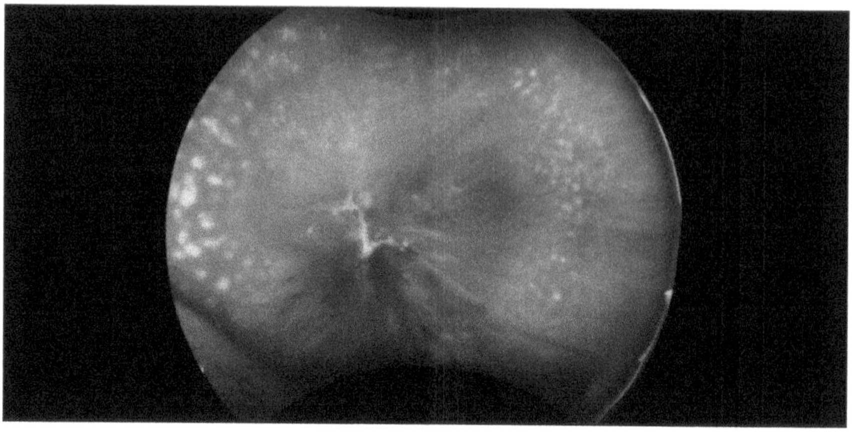

Fig. 16.13 **Case 4:** Two weeks after LIO treatment and Lucentis injection. The patient complains about visual acuity decrease

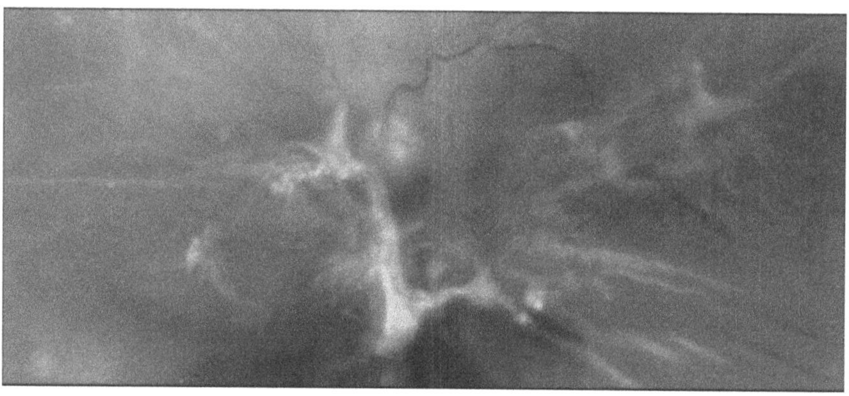

Fig. 16.14 **Case 4:** Two weeks after Avastin injection. The macula has detached. An immediate vitrectomy is scheduled

VA (RE): 0.4; subhyaloidal hemorrhage without involvement of macula.

VA (LE): HM; extensive subhyaloidal hemorrhage. The vitreous body was detached with exception of a central attachment to the temporal inferior arcade with retinal dragging (Fig. 16.16, **case 5**). Both eyes were not pretreated with laser or anti-VEGF.

First surgery

Bilateral Phaco + Avastin.

The phacoemulsification was uneventful and a vitrectomy was scheduled.

One month later: Second surgery

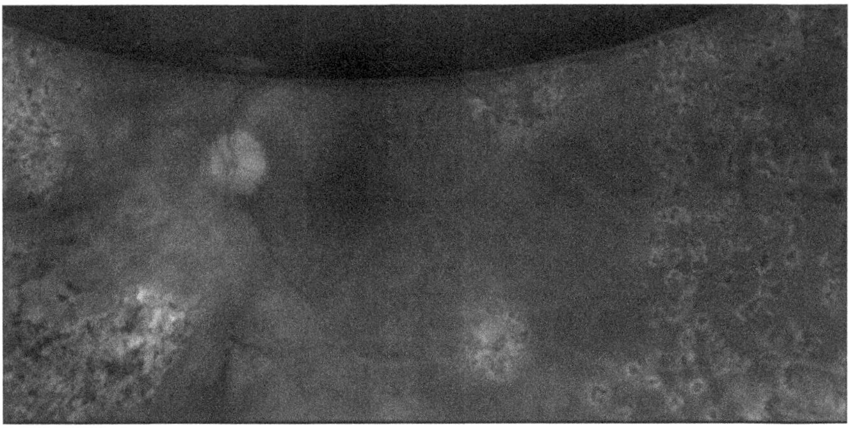

Fig. 16.15 **Case 4:** Three weeks after vitrectomy. The gas bubble is still visible

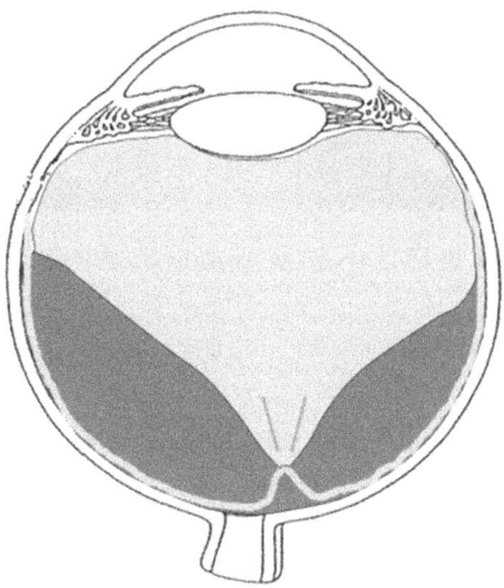

Fig. 16.16 **Case 5:** Drawing of the preoperative status of the left eye. The posterior hyaloid is detached except of one attachment to the inferior arcade. The space between retina and posterior hyaloid is filled with blood

RE: Intravitreal Avastin.

LE: PPV + peeling + laser + gas (Fig. 16.17, **case 5**).

1-month follow-up

VA (RE): CF; Vitreous hemorrhage.

VA (LE): −1.5sf = 0.6.

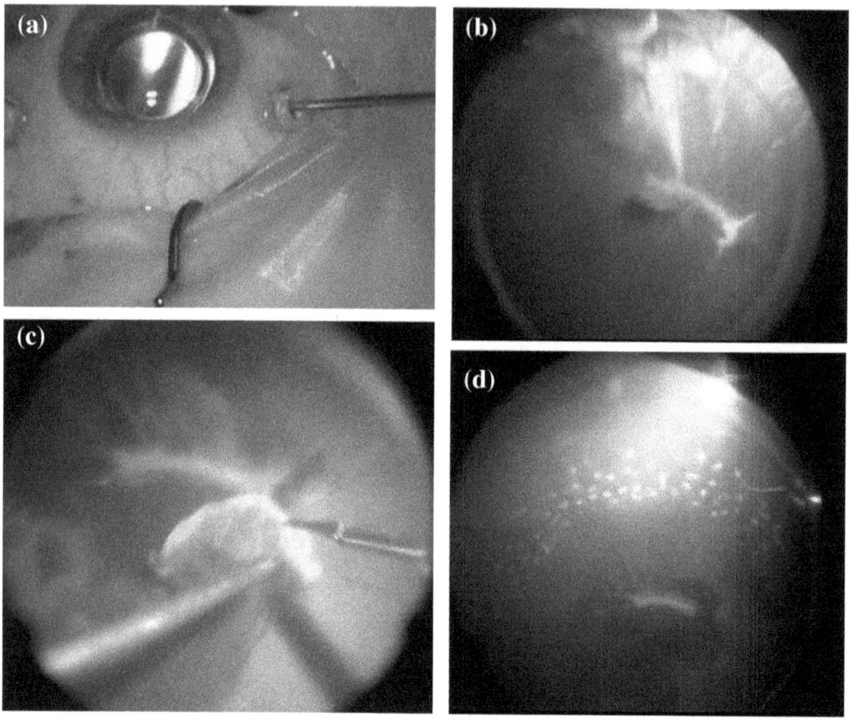

Fig. 16.17 **Case 5:** (a), We perform a stepwise surgery. Note the pseudophakic eye and the quiet anterior chamber. (b), Intraoperative image of the left eye. The vitreous gel contains no blood. Note the extensive subhyaloidal haemorrhage.(c) The left hand holds a Charles flute needle and the right hand a straight scissors. (d), PRP in a previous untreated eye. Postoperative VA = 0.6

One week before the scheduled vitrectomy on the RE the patient passed away due to a myocardial infarct.

With a hindsight of 20/20 would you have done things differently?

No. The indication for surgery was correct. The subhyaloidal hemorrhage did not resorb on its own and the adhesion of the posterior hyaloid to the retina had to be removed. In order to reduce surgical trauma, I performed a two step surgery with phaco and Avastin and 1 month later vitrectomy. The main problem with this patient was that a general anesthesia was not possible and that he could no lie still longer than 30–45 minutes. This was another reason why a stepwise procedure was chosen.

The surgical video of this case is available under this link: https://youtu.be/wNueV3Z1ZIU.

16.2 Serbian Patients

The **former Yugoslavian** healthcare system is dominated by state hospitals. The treatment is free but due to chronic underfunding there is a huge supply gap which is only partially filled by private hospitals. The private hospitals have better equipment and the patient pays for each surgery.

Diabetic screening is practically not existent. In most of the six new countries, except in Slovenia, there is no active photo-screening for ocular complications in diabetes mellitus. There is established primary diabetes care only, where patients are advised by their physicians to go to ophthalmologists for a control every 6 months for juvenile and once a year for adult diabetics, but the rest is left to the patients themselves to organize it the best way they can or will. Patients are regularly examined by an ophthalmologist first if they are admitted to the Internal Medicine Department to treat other diabetes complications. It is not rare that they have then already developed proliferative diabetic retinopathy, which is confirmed for the first time by that examination. Since proliferative diabetic retinopathy starts in the peripheral retina, it is very likely that patients themselves will search for an ophthalmological examination first when they notice that complications of retinopathy have occurred, such as vitreous hemorrhage or tractional retinal detachment that involves the macula.

The treatment planning for these Serbian cases is different compared to the Swedish patients. Why? The treatment planning is determined by local factors such as reimbursement of the surgery or the travel distance to the hospital. If the costs of the surgery are covered by the national health system and the patient lives close by then you, as a surgeon, have much more freedom for treatment planning. If the travel distance is long then the pretreatment must be done at the home clinic. We ask the home clinic to perform an anti-VEGF injection and schedule a vitrectomy 1 month later.

Sixth case report: Advanced PDR with vitreous hemorrhage; stepwise surgery
22 y/o female patient with diabetes mellitus type 1, completely missed in diabetes screening until TRD occurred; admitted to the clinic for the treatment of advanced PDR with vitreous hemorrhage, tractional retinal detachment and big submacular hemorrhage in her RE; never treated with any laser in that eye before the surgery. The visual acuity in the LE was 0.6, with already present severe PDR. Laser PRP was started in the LE in her hometown and was completed between surgeries of the RE in our clinic.

She underwent three surgeries in the RE in a stepwise procedure; **the first step** was combined phaco/vitrectomy with removal of vitreous hemorrhage, PRP to the peripheral retina, which was still attached, intravitreal Lucentis injection and air tamponade (Fig. 16.18, **case 6**). **The second step** was performed 1 week after the first surgery with en bloc excision of all visible proliferations, endodrainage of subretinal blood, completing of endolaser PRP and silicone oil 1300 cSt tamponade (Fig. 16.19, **case 6**). After 3 months, the silicone oil was successfully removed.

The preoperative visual acuity in the RE was HM and a month after silicone oil removal was CF at 1 m. The retina was completely attached but very ischemic.

The surgical videos of this case are available under this link: Two videos are available: https://youtu.be/FhPp4FqriI0 and https://youtu.be/BOe8bgFSlao.

Seventh case report: Advanced PDR with tractional retinal detachment
A 53 y/o female patient with diabetes mellitus type 1. Admitted to the clinic for the treatment of advanced PDR with tractional retinal detachment and vitreous hemorrhage in her RE. Treated before with incomplete laser PRP in both eyes. The visual acuity in the LE was 0.7.

She underwent a combined phaco/vitrectomy with en bloc excision of all visible proliferations, completed with extended endolaser PRP up to ora serrata and silicone oil 1300 cSt tamponade (Figs. 16.20 and 16.21, **case 7**). The preoperative visual acuity in the RE was CF at 2 m and the postoperative a month after surgery was 0.2. The retina was completely attached. The patient is scheduled for a silicone oil removal in 2 months.

The surgical videos of this case are available under this link: https://youtu.be/LNEvbtqQCRo.

Eighth case report: Severe PDR
A 63 y/o female patient with diabetes mellitus type 1 and history of coronary by-pass was admitted to the clinic for the treatment of severe PDR with retinal tractions in her right eye (RE). She was treated before with incomplete laser panretinal photocoagulation (PRP) in both eyes. The visual acuity in the RE was CF and LE was 0.3.

She underwent on the RE a combined phaco/vitrectomy with en bloc excision of all visible proliferations, completed with dense PRP up to the ora serrata and then air tamponade (Fig. 16.22, **case 8**). The preoperative visual acuity in the RE was CF at 2 m and the best corrected postoperative visual acuity 6 months after surgery was 0.2. The retina was completely attached.

The surgical video of this case is available under this link: https://youtu.be/FFr1KKwbsBE.

Ninth case report: Severe PDR
A 48 y/o male patient with diabetes mellitus type 1 was admitted to the clinic for the treatment of severe PDR with vitreous hemorrhage in his right eye (RE). He was treated before with almost complete PRP in that eye. The left eye (LE) was lost in neovascular glaucoma secondary to PDR with no LP.

He underwent two surgeries in RE with 3-month interval. The first was combined phaco/vitrectomy with en bloc excision of all visible proliferations, extended endolaser PRP up to ora serrata and silicone oil 1300 cSt injection (Fig. 16.23, **case 9**). After 3 months, the silicone oil was successfully removed. The preoperative visual acuity in the RE was CF at 2 m and the best corrected postoperative visual acuity 3 months after silicone oil removal was 0.1. The retina was completely attached.

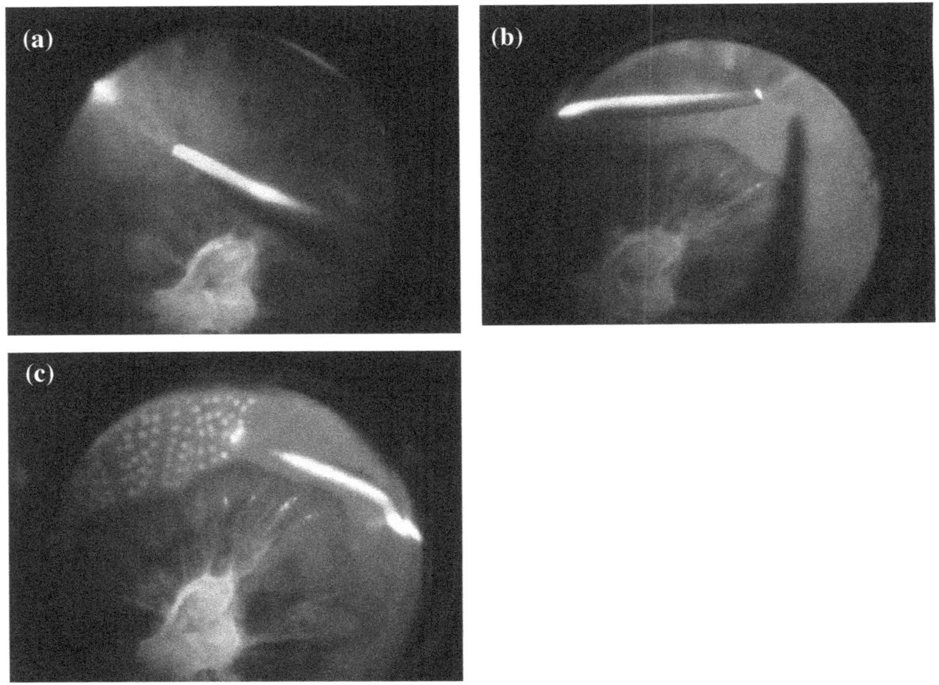

Fig. 16.18 **Case 6:** (a), Stepwise surgery in an eye with advanced PDR and vitreous hemorrhage. The retina is not pretreated with laser photocoagulation. This is the first surgery. (b), First surgery: A posterior hyaloid rhexis has been performed. (c) First surgery: A PRP from the membranes to the ora serrata. Note that the eye is not pretreated

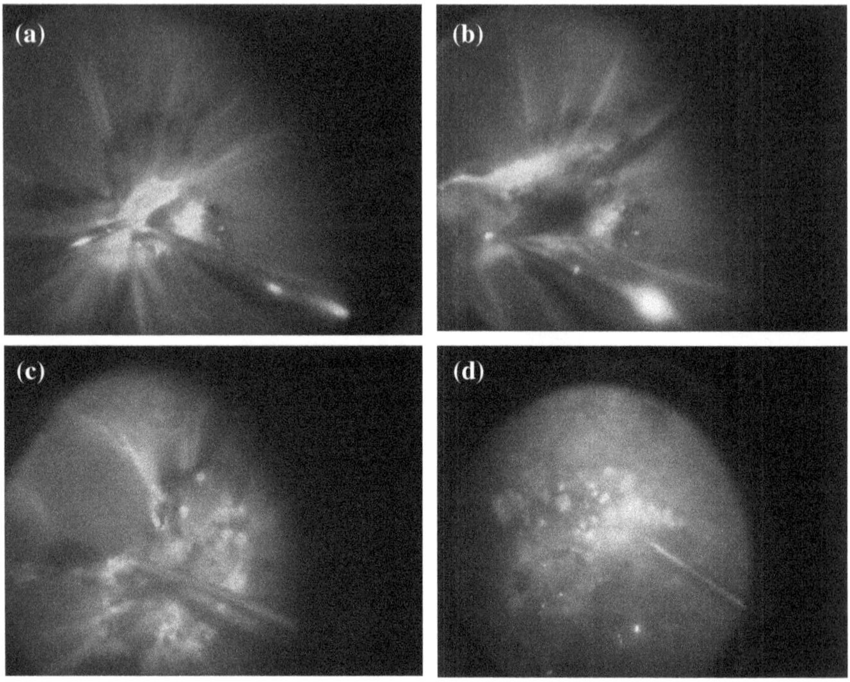

Fig. 16.19 **Case 6:** (a), Second surgery one week later: Bimanual removal of membranes. Note the central funnel. (b), Second surgery: Left hand 23G endgripping forceps and right hand knob spatula. (c) Second surgery: The membrane is removed, the funnel opened and hemostasis performed.(d), Second surgery: The retina is centrally attached and a fill-in PRP performed. The surgery is finished with a silicone oil tamponade

The surgical video of this case is available under this link: https://youtu.be/UA5mhE1l7O4.

Tenth case report: Advanced PDR with tractional retinal detachment

A 40 y/o male patient with diabetes mellitus type 1 was admitted to the clinic for the treatment of advanced PDR with tractional retinal detachment (TRD) in his LE. He was treated before with incomplete laser PRP in both eyes. The visual acuity in the RE was 0.1.

He underwent two surgeries in the LE with 4-month interval; the first was combined phaco/vitrectomy with en bloc excision of all visible proliferations, completed with dense PRP up to the ora serrata and silicone oil 1300 cSt tamponade (Figs. 16.24 and 16.25, **case 10)**. After 4 months, the silicone oil was successfully removed. The preoperative visual acuity in the LE was hand movements (HM) and the best corrected postoperative visual acuity 6 months after silicone oil removal was CF at 4 m. The retina was completely attached.

The surgical video of this case is available under this link: https://youtu.be/9yg4e6P7nkU.

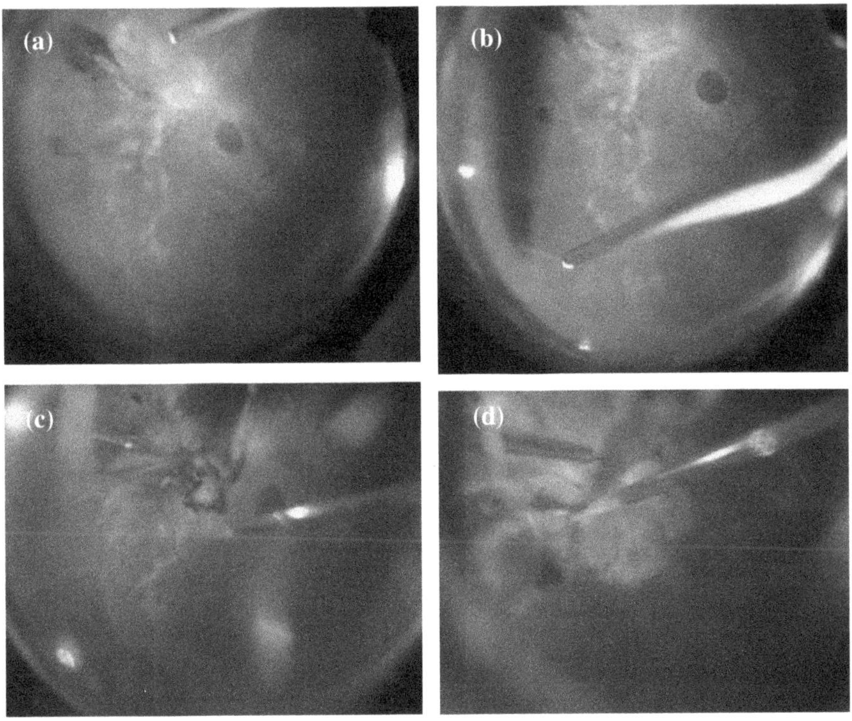

Fig. 16.20 **Case 7:** (a), An advanced PDR with attached posterior hyaloid and without laser treatment. (b), Attempt to open the peripheral posterior hyaloid.(c), Bimanual delamination of the peripheral posterior hyaloid. (d), The white tissue to the right is posterior hyaloid, the underlying tissue is retina

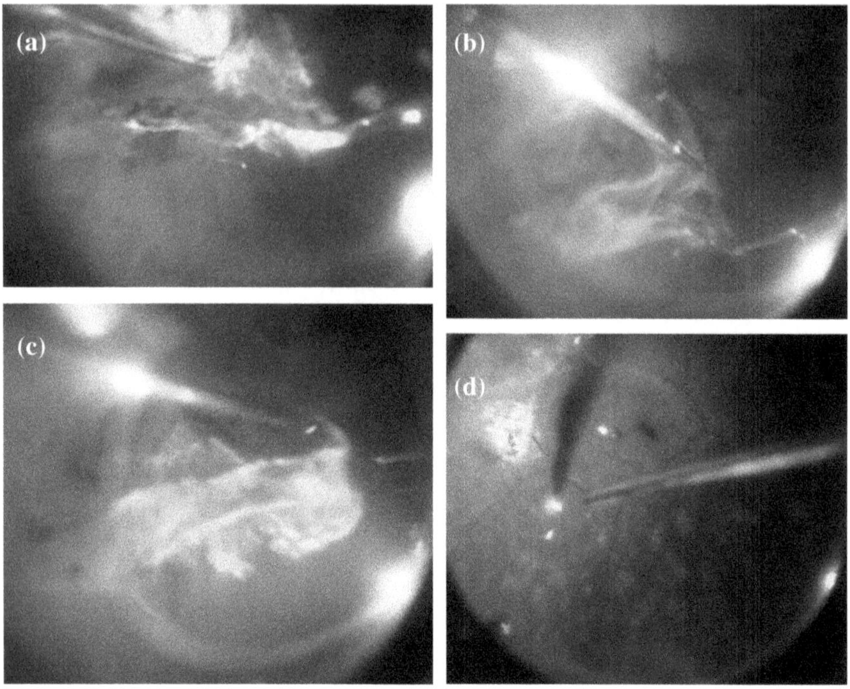

Fig. 16.21 **Case 7:** (a), Delamination of posterior hyaloid with knob spatula (left) and intravitreal forceps (right). (b), Delamination of posterior hyaloid at the inferonasal quadrant. (c), The posterior hyaloid has to be removed up to the vitreous base. This is very time consuming. (d), After complete removal of the posterior hyaloid a PRP is performed. The case is closed with 1300 cSt silicone oil

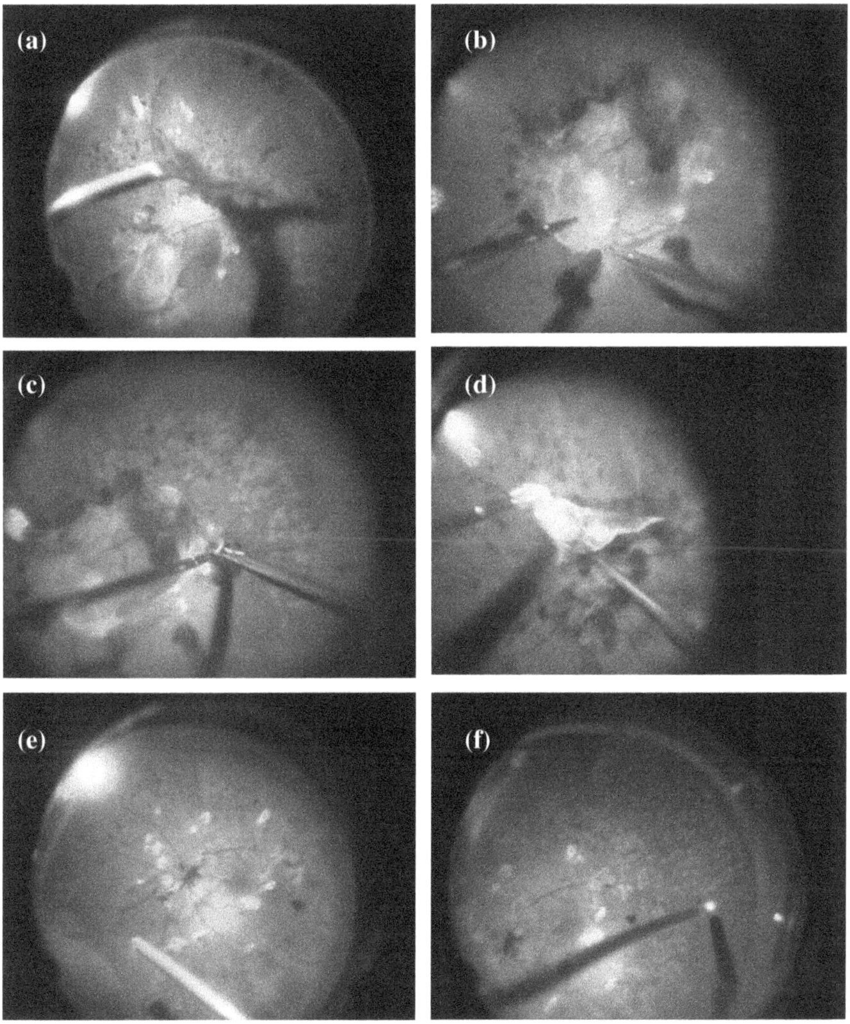

Fig. 16.22 **Case 8:** (a), Induction of a peripheral PVD in an eye with severe PDR. (b), A posterior hyaloid rhexis has been performed. The next step is the delamination of the central posterior hyaloid. (c), Bimanual delamination of preretinal membranes. (d), The membranes are almost removed. Note the retinal bleedings. (e), The retinal bleedings have been cauterized. The next step is a shaving of the vitreous base. (f), A PRP from the arcades to the ora serrata

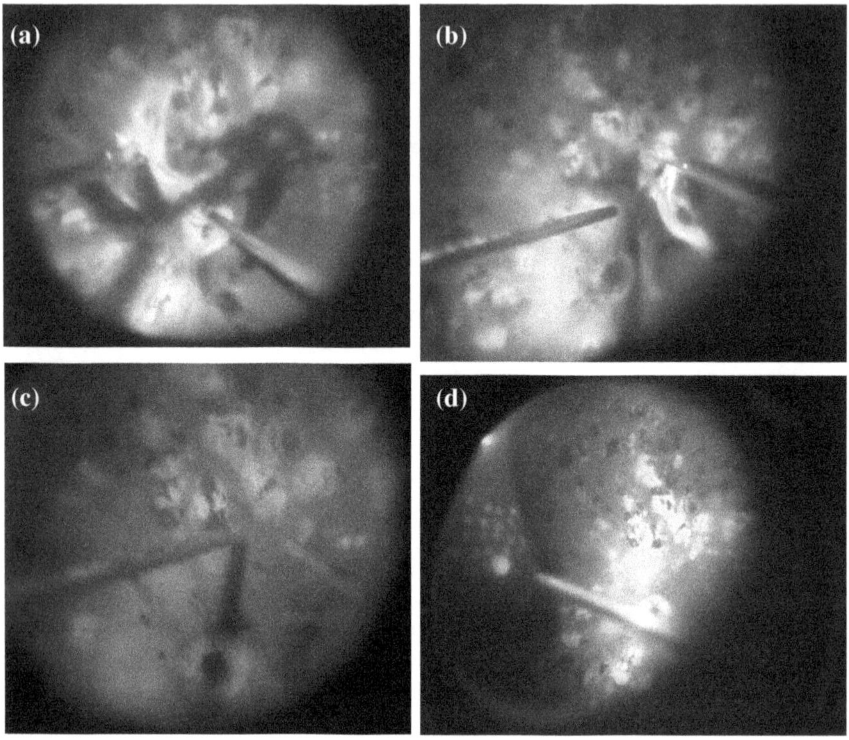

Fig. 16.23 **Case 9:** (a), A laser treated retina with central membranes. The removal of membranes is followed of retinal bleedings. (b), Removal of the delaminated membrane with the vitreous cutter. (c), Endodiathermy of retinal bleedings. (d), Fill-in PRP up to the ora serrata which is simple with bimanual technique. This case is much easier because the retina has been pretreated

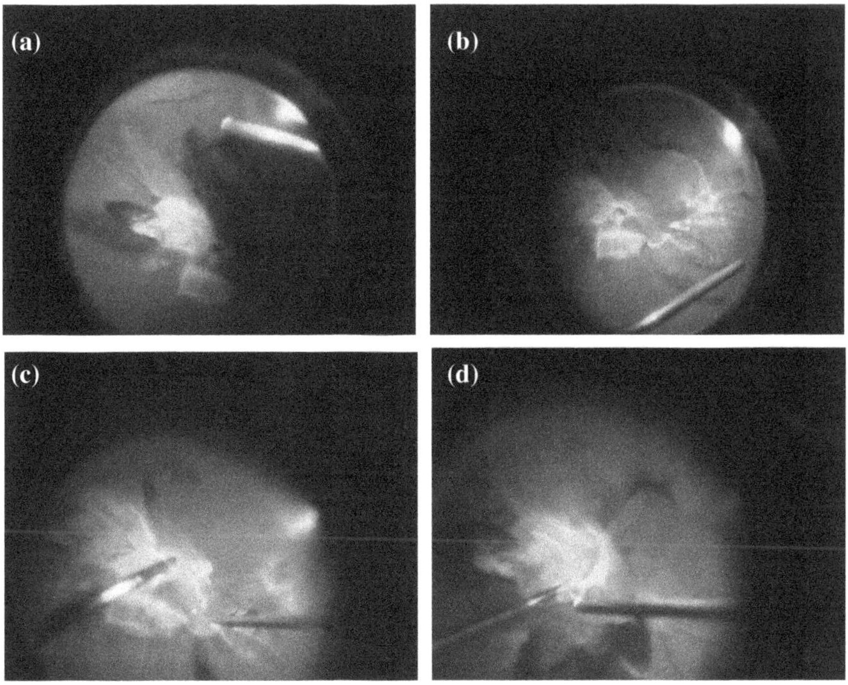

Fig. 16.24 **Case 10:** (a), Partial tractional retinal detachment with central membranes.(b) A posterior hyaloid rhexis. The opening in the posterior hyaloid is well visible. (c), Bimanual delamination of preretinal membranes. (d), Removal of delaminated membranes with vitreous cutter

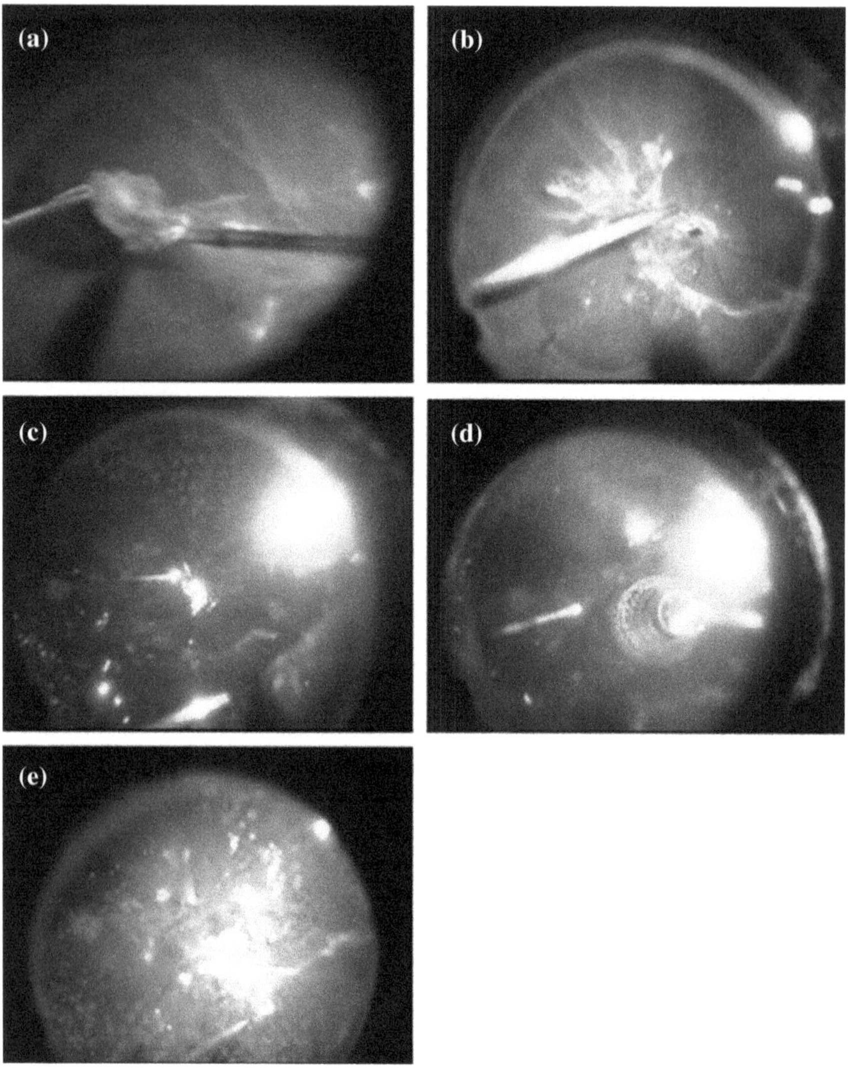

Fig. 16.25 **Case 10:** (a) Final delamination of membranes with straight scissors. (b), Injection of PFCL to reattach the retina. (c), PRP up to the ora serrata with bimanual technique. (d), Injection of 1300 cSt silicone oil. (e), A completely attached retina under silicone oil

Surgical Materials

(In alphabetical order):

BSS Plus®: Alcon. Indication: Lens-sparing vitrectomy.

C_2F_6: Many Providers, for Example, Alcon

C_3F_8: Many Providers, for Example, Alcon

Caliper of CASTROVIEJO Geuder No.: 19135

Cannula, 23G for injection of dye: DORC 1281.A5D06.

Cannula, 25G for injection of dye: MedOne. Ref. 3225 or DORC 1272.SD25.

Cannula, double-barrel injection Dual bore 23-gauge cannula for injection of PFCL. DORC: EFD.06.

Capsular tension ring with injector: CROMA, DORC, Morcher, Arcadophta.

Celoftal® (for cornea): Alcon.

Chandelier light in trocar: ALCON: Chandelier Accurus 8065751574 or Chandelier Constellation 8065751577; DORC: 23-gauge Chandelier light 3269.EB06 and Synergetics 25G Awh Chandelier. 56.51.23P or 56.51.25P

Chandelier light in sclera: 27-gauge twinlight from Eckhardt 3269.MBD27; Synergetics: 25-Gauge Awh Chandelier 56.20.25.

Contact Lens, Plano. Indication: Macular peeling. DORC: Disposable vitrectomy lens: Flat. 1284.DD

Ocucoat® (lubrication of cornea): Bausch & Lomb.

Silicone oil 1000cSt: Fluoron. G-80 710, DORC or Bausch & Lomb

Silicone oil 5000cSt: Fluoron. G-80 810

U. Spandau and Z. Tomic, *Small-Gauge Vitrectomy for Diabetic Retinopathy*,
https://doi.org/10.1007/978-3-031-26204-3

Silicone oil cannula, 23-gauge: Med One: 3241st PolyTip Cannula 23-gauge 10 mm (Sanisoglu) or DORC: 1272.VFI06. 23-gauge 7 mm

SF_6: many providers, for example, Alcon.

Trocar forceps for the removal of trocars. DORC. 1278.

Valved Trocar System by Alcon: 23G, 8065751657

Valved Trocar System by DORC: 23G, 1272.ED206.

Valved Trocar System by Geuder: 23G, G 33 445

Valved Trocar System by Oertli: 23G, Autoseal PMS®

Dyes:

Brilliant Peel®: (Brilliant Blue G). Indication: Staining of ILM. Geuder, Heidelberg

Membrane Blue®: (Trypan blue). Indication: Staining of vitreous and epiretinal membranes. DORC

Membrane BlueDual®: (Trypan blue + Brilliant Blue G). Indication: Staining of vitreous and epiretinal membranes and ILM. DORC.

Monoblue®: (Trypan blue). Indication: Staining of vitreous and epiretinal membranes. Arcadophta, Toulouse, France

Triamcinolone acetonide (Volon A®): Indication: Staining of vitreous and epiretinal membranes. Pfizer.

19 Companies

Alcon
Alcon Laboratories (U.K.) Ltd.
Pentagon Park
Boundary Way
Hemel Hempstead
Herts HP2 7UD, England
Phone: 44+1442.341.234
www.alcon.com

Arcadophta
293, route de Seysses
F-31100 Toulouse
Phone: 0033/561/405235
Fax: 0033/5617 408 466
info@arcadophta.com
www.arcadophta.com

Bausch & Lomb
United Kingdom
Europe, Middle East and Africa Division European Headquarters
Bausch & Lomb House
106-114 London Road
Kingston-Upon-Thames
Surrey KT2 6QJ, England
Phone: 44-20-8781-5500
Fax: 44-20-8781-2989
www.bausch.com

U. Spandau and Z. Tomic, *Small-Gauge Vitrectomy for Diabetic Retinopathy*, https://doi.org/10.1007/978-3-031-26204-3

DORC
Dutch Ophthalmic Research
Center International BV
Scheijdelveweg 2
3214 VN Zuidland
The Netherlands
Phone: +31 181 458080
Fax: +31 181 458090
www.dorc.nl

Ellex Services Europe
La Chaufferie
555 chemin du bois
69140 Rillieux la Pape France
Phone: +33 4 82 91 04 60

Ellex Deutschland GmbH
Edisonstraße 20
63512 Hainburg
Phone: +49 6182 829 6900

Eye Technology Ltd.
19 Totman Crescent
Brook Road Industrial Estate
Rayleigh
Essex SS6 7UY
United Kingdom
sales@eye-tech.co.uk

Fluoron GmbH
Magirus-Deutz-Strasse 10
89077 Ulm
Phone: 0731/20 559 970
Fax: 0731/205 599 728
info@fluoron.de
www.fluoron.de

Geuder AG
Hertzstr. 4
69126 Heidelberg,
Phone: 06221/3066
Fax: 06221/303 122
info@geuder.de
www.geuder.de

IRIDEX Corporation
1212 Terra Bella Avenue
Mountain View, CA 94,043, USA
www.iridex.com

MedOne Surgical Inc.
Sarasota, FL USA 34 243
www.MedOne.com

Oculus, Inc. GmbH
Münchholzhäuser 29 st
D-35582 Wetzlar
Phone: 0641/20 050
Fax: 0641/2005255
sales@oculus.de
www.oculus.de

Oertli Instrumente AG
Hafnerwisenstr. 4
CH-9442 Berneck,
Tel: 0041/71/74742 2000
Fax 0041/71/74742 90
E-mail: info@oertli-instruments.com
www.oertli-instruments.com

Ophtec BV
Schweitzerlaan 15
9728 NR Groningen,
Netherlands
www.ophtec.com

Synergetics France GmbH
Synergetics France SARL
6 Place de la Madeleine
75008 Paris
France
Phone: 825 825 250
Fax: 1 64 11 16 99
E-mail: plecharpentier@synergeticsusa.com
www.synergeticsusa.com

Index

U. Spandau and Z. Tomic, *Small-Gauge Vitrectomy for Diabetic Retinopathy*,
https://doi.org/10.1007/978-3-031-26204-3

GPSR Compliance
The European Union's (EU) General Product Safety Regulation (GPSR) is a set of rules that requires consumer products to be safe and our obligations to ensure this.

If you have any concerns about our products, you can contact us on

ProductSafety@springernature.com

In case Publisher is established outside the EU, the EU authorized representative is:

Springer Nature Customer Service Center GmbH
Europaplatz 3
69115 Heidelberg, Germany

www.ingramcontent.com/pod-product-compliance
Ingram Content Group UK Ltd.
Pitfield, Milton Keynes, MK11 3LW, UK
UKHW021457031026
15588UKWH00002B/859
* 9 7 8 3 0 3 1 2 6 2 0 5 0 *